Menopause
Bootcamp

Menopause Bootcamp

Optimize Your Health,
Empower Your Self,
and Flourish as You Age

Suzanne Gilberg-Lenz, MD

With Marjorie Korn

HARPER WAVE

An Imprint of HarperCollins*Publishers*

This book contains advice and information relating to health care. It should be used to supplement rather than replace the advice of your doctor or another trained health professional. If you know or suspect you have a health problem, it is recommended that you seek your physician's advice before embarking on any medical program or treatment. All efforts have been made to assure the accuracy of the information contained in this book as of the date of publication. This publisher and the author disclaim liability for any medical outcomes that may occur as a result of applying the methods suggested in this book.

FIRST EDITION

Library of Congress Cataloging-in-Publication Data has been applied for.

ISBN 978-0-06-314318-0

22 23 24 25 26   LSC   10 9 8 7 6 5 4 3 2 1

Thank you to my third grade teacher, Miss Creigh. You were right.

"*The one person who will never leave us, whom we will never lose, is ourself. Learning to love our female selves is where our search for love must begin.*"

—bell hooks

"*Every beginning is only a sequel, after all, and the book of events is always open halfway through.*"

—Wislawa Szymborska

CONTENTS

Introduction

Some profound journeys begin in a patient's
room that's adorned with Tibetan prayer
flags. Others start at the hair salon.

I want to tell you about something that I'm still trying to process. Two years ago, I decided to stop coloring my hair. I won't lie, it was no act of feminist defiance of beauty standards—at least not at first. I was tired of spending so much time and money getting my hair done. And for the record, this was two years before covid-19 forced a bunch of people to embrace their gray. I had hatched a plan with my hairdresser, who's been a dear friend for fifteen years, to have one last fling: I'd dye my auburn hair a bright shade of blond, then allow it to go gray. So I was sitting in the chair, and he started mixing up a pot of chestnut hair coloring *without my permission*. When I questioned him about it, he said, "You're not ready." I was dumbfounded. I'm not ready? Says who?

What he was really saying was that I needed to keep up the ruse of youth and it was his job as my friend to help me do so. To him, and to a lot of other people, having gray hair is like saying "Hi, I'm Suzanne, and I'm an old woman." And of course, I'm not. I maintain a thriving private practice. I still feel passion. I give interviews and run bootcamps and consider myself an activist for the causes I believe in. But gray = old, and it's all downhill from there. Listen, it wasn't just him. Everyone seemed to have an opinion on my damn hair: friends, colleagues, even patients. They weren't trying to be mean. I think they were honestly confused. The comments were underpinned by a question: Why wouldn't you want to look younger? The women in their sixties and seventies were the most befuddled. It was as if the subterfuge works only if we are all pretending together. Now more than ever before, to look your age is to break the rules—and not in a good way. Think about that for a minute. I'm an ob-gyn who's attended the births of thousands of babies and raised two of her own. There's no way I could be thirty. I needed all fifty-five of my years to get to where I am. And now I do embrace my gray as an act of feminist resistance—not to mention that it is a huge time-saver and I have better things to do with my money. There's more to unpack, and you came here to talk about menopause, not my hair. I'll just say one more thing: If I have learned anything in my fifty-five years, it's that women are expected to look and behave in a certain way. And letting our hair go gray means "letting ourselves go"; in other words, owning our actual age is seen as some sort of defeat or lack of interest in our beauty.

Talking about menopause is like letting our gray grow in. For many of us it's scary, an admission that we're not young anymore. That's one of the major reasons, I believe, that we don't talk about it. But that silence comes at a huge cost to both our health and our ability to live fully in our bodies. So right now, in these pages, we're going to start to change that. *Menopause Bootcamp* is going to educate you on what happens in your body during the menopausal transition and afterward. We'll learn about the symptoms and the solutions, including both the latest research and evidence-based wellness practices. And we'll explore ways in which you can make this time of life feel authentic and joyful.

The fact that we're here discussing menopause is in itself a small act of rebellion. Until very recently, few of us talked about it in public, even though millions of women are going through some stage of it right now. How much do *you* discuss it? Sure, it's not really dinner party conversation, but at least it should be fair game with your friends. After two decades of practice, I can tell you that there are women who won't talk about it with their closest friends. Or with their own mothers and daughters. It can even be hard for them to bring it up with their doctors.

Before we continue, I want to make a quick note about pronouns. Throughout this book I refer to both "women" and "people" when describing those who are going through the menopause transition. Some people going through menopause are cis women, meaning that they were assigned female at birth and identify as a woman. Likewise, people across the gender spectrum can experience menopause. Hence my effort to use language to invite all people into this journey. And although my solution to pronouns may be inelegant (I sent the book's copy editor a basket of muffins), I hope you'll find it to be respectful and inclusive.

Menopause Bootcamp is about hoisting up the big tent that covers all of us. Our experiences with our symptoms and our life conditions are unique, but there are overriding societal winds that encircle all of us. In addition to recognizing yourself in this book, I hope you will also acknowledge the experiences of others. Our common denominator? We've all got highs, and we've all got lows. This is not lip service; we're going to see one another through them, together.

I hope my authentic interest and recognition of our similarities and differences is also a reason why my patients feel comfortable enough to speak about their concerns with me. They feel seen and their experiences validated. Over the past few years, I've become something of a menopause guru. I think that's because I'm always interested in whatever no one else is into. Dry vagina? Check! Painful sex? Check! Leaking urine? Check! When a patient comes to me with a problem I'm not up on, I go out and learn more about it. Because if it's happening to her, it's happening to a lot of people. It feeds my endless curiosity about the human experience.

But to get there—to be able to talk about vaginal tissue and sex drive and skin changes—we have to convince women to trust that doctors care about their overall well-being. That seems like Doctoring 101, right? Well, the medical system has a long and disgusting history of overlooking, ignoring, and manipulating women. Research studies have for decades not included women in their pool of test subjects, which means that for years we've been subjected to treatments whose safety and efficacy have been proven only for men. There haven't even been enough studies on women's health issues themselves. There are predatory doctors and others shilling bullshit products. And inferior care *especially* happens to older folks, people of color, those across the gender spectrum, and persons with disabilities, among others.

For all those reasons, I created a Menopause Bootcamp series in southern California, where I live and practice, in which a group of women get together to learn about the changes their bodies are undergoing, hear about a wide variety of solutions, share their experiences, and gain a sense of community. If you can't make it to one, this book will give you all the information and tools you need to help empower your life.

Oftentimes, we start out with identifying goals. I have a few myself: to demystify how the transition actually occurs, to give women information they need to make better decisions about their bodies, and to dispel the pernicious belief that menopause is an ending. It's not. For many, it is a new beginning.

Before we get into some of the reasons why I believe this weird taboo around being postmenopausal exists, let's lay out a few facts. The median age of menopause onset is 51.4 years, but the menopause transition typically begins eight to ten years before that. Clinically speaking, you are in menopause when your period has been absent for twelve consecutive months. In that way, it's straightforward. What makes this time unique is that the symptoms are different for every person going through it.

Menopause Bootcamp is designed to help you understand what's happening with your body and go over ways in which this transition may be unique to you. Every so often, a patient tells me that they feel as though menopause is punishment for being born with a uterus. I understand why it can feel that way sometimes. Let's take a quick run through all the ways that menopause can upturn a person's life. Of course, there are the hot flashes that come on out of nowhere and can make you feel as though you have entered a sauna. Eighty-five percent of women go through this, and they can last from two to ten years— and 9 percent of women over seventy experience occasional hot flashes! Show of hands from those of you who have sleep problems. They can take several forms: trouble falling asleep, trouble staying asleep, waking up from night sweats, or needing to get up to go to the bathroom several times per night. There are hair loss and skin changes, not to mention mood changes and depression. Plus there are sexual changes, such as vaginal dryness and decreased sex drive. Because who wants to have penetrative sex or masturbate if it hurts?

I'm here to tell you that there are things you can do—both medical and lifestyle changes—that will make this transition easier. After all, if your period stops in your late forties or early fifties and you live to see your eighties (the average American woman's life expectancy is 80.5 years), you'll spend between a third and half of your life in menopause. And we are developing a more nuanced understanding of what's going on to help you manage your symptoms better. Do we know everything there is to know about menopause? No. Science has a lot of catching up to do. But even now, there are medicines and treatments that are safe for many women. And there are a host of ways to make menopause more manageable that don't come from Walgreens.

The question that is always asked at the top of the hour concerns menopausal hormone therapy (MHT). And yes, it's a hot-button issue. You may have even made up your mind that it's not for you, perhaps because you've heard that it increases your risk of developing cancer. The science is actually more nuanced than that, and there are women for whom MHT is safe and effective. We'll go into the pros and cons, and then it'll be up to you and your physician as to whether it seems like a good option. With few exceptions, I'm not trying to advocate for any one intervention. There's no one-size-fits-all solution when it comes to menopause. But it's important to know the menu of options.

Western medicine has its limitations. Part of those are what I mentioned before—that academic medical research, which produces the majority of findings, has a pattern of neglecting women. A 2013 survey conducted by the John Hopkins University School of Medicine in Baltimore found that out of more than five hundred obstetrics and gynecology residents—that is, doctors with a focus on *women's* health—67 percent reported having limited knowledge about why menopause symptoms occur, 68 percent didn't know enough about hormone therapy, and a whopping 72 percent needed to learn more about cardiovascular disease. This is a particularly ominous statistic given that heart disease is the number one killer of women and there are interventions that postmenopausal women should be doing to keep themselves (and their tickers) healthy. Most ob-gyns don't feel equipped to deal with menopause. For most of them, here's what happens: As a doctor, you want to feel that you can help people. So if you know that you don't have the answers to certain medical problems, you might not ask the questions.

We're learning more and more from women's stories and from research that doctors have a pattern of not taking a woman's needs or her pain seriously. Beyond that, Western medicine has other limitations. It's based around diagnosing and treating diseases—not people. And it leaves huge holes in the system. Think of Dr. House, who in every episode of the eponymous TV series was presented with a case no one else could figure out. He and his team often uncovered the solution in some arcane medical text or case study. And with eight minutes left in the episode, House would have his *aha!* moment, prescribe the exact right course of treatment, and stick the patient file in a drawer. Case closed.

The real world doesn't usually operate like that. Patients often have a variety of issues going on at once that require different interventions and continued care. And we know that there is a strong mind-body connection and that neglecting to acknowledge the person and focusing only on the issue is a dangerous habit. The real world doesn't wrap human conditions up in a neat package with a bow. People evolve. Symptoms come and go. Perceptions change. Care must be ongoing, nimble, and responsive to changes in a person's situation.

I understood the limitations to the disease-first approach from the time I started medical school at the University of Southern California. Perhaps it was because I had a winding path getting there. I went from studying art history at Wesleyan University and thinking I was bad at math* to working with severely emotionally disturbed children in

---

* That belief started as a bad grade in middle school geometry. It was only when I was doing a postbaccalaureate premed program at the renowned women's school Mills College in Oakland, California, that I realized I am, in fact, great at math. I aced the most detested class, organic chemistry, and not only that, I loved the class! It was then that I realized I'd been conditioned to keep my intellect a secret, for fear of outshining the boys in my elementary and middle school classes. The patriarchy starts infiltrating our minds at a young age, and it wasn't until I attended an all-women's school that I realized the lie that I was living.

a group home in San Francisco to finally heeding my call to become a doctor. That decision was a combination of pathological idealism, a need to serve, intense curiosity, and a love of humans in all their complex messiness.

USC taught me the inner workings of the body, and I am grateful for that. But I often felt that my mostly male colleagues didn't fully appreciate the fact that cis women are not just guys with vaginas. Yet the idea that what separates us is simply genitalia is pervasive in medicine. Yes, there have been hard-won advancements in the field of women's health, and we owe a debt of gratitude to the women who came before us, took part in studies (sometimes, tragically, not of their own volition), and taught us so much about the female body and how it works—and what happens when things "break." But to me, that toggle switch of working-versus-broken neglects something critical: that women are not simply an amalgam of ovaries, uterus, breasts. They're a whole person, and it's only when you treat the whole person that you can provide the best care possible. Which is why, with certain patients who are interested in it, I refer them to acupuncturists or other practitioners of complementary and alternative medicine. (I also explore Ayurvedic medicine, a practice that's thousands of years old and is based on the idea that for a body to be healthy, there needs to be an integration of body, mind, and spirit.) My patients are often surprised that in addition to counseling them on topics such as mammograms and vaginal dryness, I offer recommendations such as meditation, exercise, acupuncture, and specific herbs for PMS and hot flashes.

Complementary medicine instructs us to consider the whole person. That's how we should be thinking about the menopause transition. It has another edge over Western medicine, which has a hyperfocus on identifying what's "wrong." Think about it like this: A woman comes to me with a laundry list of issues. She can't sleep, and she's gaining weight. She's still getting her period, but she's begun to feel as though she's out of sync with her body. Pretty often, she asks if it could be a thyroid issue. She wants it to be something that's fixable. We can run a blood test and check her thyroid, but nine times out of ten it's normal. The likely explanation is that she's in perimenopause. Which means that the issues she's telling me about aren't a sign that something is *wrong*. What she's describing is normal—yet it can be really uncomfortable, both physically and emotionally. We can do things to help manage her symptoms so they don't drive her crazy, but we need to get out of the mindset that something is the matter. It's not. Menopause is normal and nothing to be ashamed of.

This leads me to another goal of *Menopause Bootcamp*. I want us all to dismantle the stigma around this time of life. In other societies, older people are revered, as age confers wisdom and endurance. "Old" in this country means fragile. Unattractive. *Dried up*—and, yes, that's laden with sexual connotations, largely negative ones. This is not just a problem that women are facing, either; men are also pushed aside owing to their age, and they have to deal with their own bodily changes. But I contend that the effects are more pernicious among women.

Listen, I practice medicine in Beverly Hills, which is ground zero of the absolutely insane notion that only women who are *young* are worthy of our attention and attraction. Yes, I sometimes find myself jealous when I see a tiny twentysomething in yoga pants. I'm being honest here—I'm a woman in society, too, and I'm not immune to the pressures we all feel. But what I don't want to be is a person who can't let that go. And it's hard, because there are tons of messages out there telling us that our worth is based on our beauty and sexual viability—and that if we are too old to have children, we are perhaps not worth anything. If you don't know what I mean, watch the skit from the TV show *Inside Amy Schumer* called "Last F**kable Day," in which Patricia Arquette and Tina Fey are toasting Julia Louis-Dreyfus on her last day of being desirable, to be demure about it. "In every actress's life, the media decides when you finally reach the point when you're not believably f**kable anymore," Louis-Dreyfus explains. "If you shoot a sex scene before your birthday, they're like, 'Hurry up, hurry up,'" Fey adds, "because they think your vagina's going to turn into a hermit crab."

I'll take any opportunity I get to say this: women deserve to be seen and heard at every age. Our worth is not tied to our physical attractiveness or ability to bear children. That is some patriarchal *bullshit*. We are strong as individuals, and we are stronger as a community. We have the opportunity to give up our fear of vulnerability. *Menopause Bootcamp* isn't about forming a club of women who no longer shop for tampons; it's about creating a big tent occupied by people who own their bodies and their beings at every point along the way. Aging isn't something to be afraid of! We've been on the planet for a long time. We have a lot of wisdom and stories and experience. When we band together, we can really get some creative, witchy juices going. This isn't your grandma's "golden years." Your fifties don't have to be the beginning of the end.

Don't get me wrong: it's not easy to develop this mindset. It can sometimes feel downright impossible. But we all have to get there one way or another. I want to revisit that gray hair story for a moment, because it actually changed me more than I expected. Continuing to go gray has been an extended watershed moment in terms of being in my body and accepting it. It's a process that takes intense emotional effort because it comes into direct conflict with the forces instructing us, as women, to conform, to stay young. When we deny who we are, we abandon ourselves and the unique experience we deserve. I know that it's really scary and painful for some people, but it truly is so much better to be who you are. We waste so much energy on trying to be something we're not.

It doesn't have to be this way, this constant push-pull between autonomy and society. And certainly I respect every person's decision. But when we are isolated and don't talk about the choices we are making, they can become a menace. Nothing really great grows in what I call the "shade of shame." I'm here to help till the soil, give you some nutrients, and trim the branches to reveal some sunlight that will help grow whatever you want to plant.

Ultimately, this book is about empowering *you*—because I'm not a historian or an activist, but I am a doctor who treats people with uteruses, something I take very seriously. I've also been influenced by the younger generation, who want to have more open conversations about how to be body and sex positive. Menopause isn't easy, and there are some additional conditions—such as osteoporosis, cancer, and cognitive decline—that can come with the territory. Only you can navigate this time for yourself. Just remember that there are a lot of people in your corner who want to help you. Including me.

* * *

Menopause Bootcamp has been at least a decade in the making, but my path to women's advocacy started when I did my obstetrics and gynecology residency at Cedars-Sinai Medical Center in Los Angeles.

In 1997, I was a newly married thirty-year-old intern, and I did the thing you're not supposed to do as a doctor in training and *certainly* not your first year in the program: I got pregnant. The pressure was enormous. I doubled down on my work, because I didn't want to miss one second of training. I also didn't want to risk being seen as weak by my coresidents or faculty members. I will never be able to adequately describe the physical, mental, and spiritual toll residency takes; to do it while pregnant was truly painful. I had no time to adequately rest or nourish myself. I worked eighty- to one-hundred-hour weeks, was on my feet for hours at a time, ran down hallways, and pushed heavy equipment. I bent and contorted my growing body to fit at a bedside, attend a birth, or stand flush alongside the operating room table. I developed gestational diabetes, probably due to that insane lifestyle. I was barely surviving—and it's what medical training tells us to do.

The toughest and most badass residents are rewarded. I was stubborn and refused to ask for help, but the nurses looked out for me, whether it was sneaking in some orange juice with a straw under my surgical mask during a surgery so I wouldn't faint or sending me for naps in empty patient rooms. I really do not know how I made it through. I was so much stronger than I realized.

Meanwhile, I was trying to prepare for the baby's arrival. My husband and I chose a natural childbirth protocol called the Bradley Method: labor mostly at home and no epidural. I educated myself on the physiological process of labor and birth. My partner and I were confident in our comfort measures, advocacy, and consent. Delivery, we knew, is a normal human process, not a medical emergency. But that was the 1990s! Women who showed up in labor and delivery with a doula and a birth plan were mocked by the doctors and nurses. And I couldn't afford a doula anyway.

I'd been scheduled to work on my due date. The residency program director said it was because first-time mothers often miss their due date, but in looking back, I suspect that she was baiting me into giving in. And I did. I had to. I was miserable, exhausted, and enormous and told my chief resident that I needed to go on leave. I had only a week to feel bad about it before I went into labor.

And what a wild ride it was. After spending the first twelve hours at home, I rolled onto the labor and delivery floor like a banshee, moaning and thrashing—and traumatizing my coresident on call that night. One of my nurse besties came in on her day off to care for me, informing me that my cervix was only one centimeter dilated. My obstetrician was there and immediately started pushing drugs to make labor happen faster. Each intervention brought more intense pain coupled with the contractions, and I finally begged for an epidural. The birth plan that my husband and I had come up with was slipping away as medical decisions were being made outside the room by doctors—none of whom included me or asked for my consent. The interventions, though not necessarily dangerous, didn't respect the authority of my voice while in labor. It was a common occurrence then, and it still happens now.

I want to be clear here: I still count that day I met Jaron, my beautiful son, as one of the best and most transformative of my life. But over time, I came to understand that in the process of giving birth to him, I had been robbed of autonomy. In retrospect, that instilled my deep desire to always listen to my patients' lived experiences and understand their unique points of view. Twenty-three years later, I am well known in my community for always being an advocate for patients' autonomy. I support their wishes while maintaining my semi-conventional, evidence-based bona fides. Because of my resolve to listen, learn, inform, collaborate, and educate, I have been a favorite of doulas, midwives, and natural childbirth experts since I started my practice while maintaining the respect of my most conventional colleagues. Childbirth is too important to approach it any other way. As we face the crisis in health care, systemic racism, and racial disparities in medical outcomes, we must invoke and expect these principles and ideals even more fiercely. Lives literally depend on this.

I'll finish the story quickly. Two weeks after giving birth, my residency director called to let me know that she'd be unable to guarantee that my highly coveted residency spot would still be mine if I took more than six weeks of maternity leave—a threat I didn't realize was illegal until years later. A month after that, I returned to eighty- to one-hundred-hour workweeks, all while quietly living with postpartum depression for a year. And I know that some of you reading this will have been forced into a maternity leave that was even shorter than that. I'm sorry for all of us—mothers, partners, newborns, and other children in the family—who have to endure this system.

I didn't have a voice then, but I sure as hell do now. And just as giving birth is a normal (and extraordinary) human experience, so is menopause. For some of us, it can even be extraordinary. So that's why I'm highly vocal about it, too. (Also, if you haven't already noticed, I'm not shy. Don't expect a lot of euphemisms.) My practice has become a destination for women who've seen other doctors who are either prudish or undereducated about menopause, leaving them feeling frustrated and alone. I wanted to help them. Eventually, I knew, I would need to make my voice louder. And around seven years ago, I sat down to write this book.

Then I was diagnosed with breast cancer. I was only forty-seven. *Shit.* It was a low-grade tumor, so in retrospect it feels as though I didn't so much have a brush with death as I did a brush with mortality. Clinically speaking, I knew the literature and science, so I had an idea of what I needed to do. But I remember speaking to a good friend of mine who's a trauma surgeon, and his reaction summed up the prevailing notion: "Your breast is trying to kill you." It was his way of saying that I should have a mastectomy. I've heard other people say that. "Cut my breasts off, they're trying to kill me."

I never saw it that way. I saw the cancer as a thing that was happening to my body. It led me to start thinking about how I might build a relationship with my body where I didn't fear that it was trying to hurt me and actually accept it. That followed years of body image struggles similar to what others go through: worries about my looks, concerns that I was never thin or fit enough. Perhaps I had never fully dealt with those. But the threat to my body that breast cancer posed was different, not something I could ignore or sweep under the rug. I had to deal with it, so I did. That, along with the thorough lesson in control—or, more specifically, in my lack thereof—helped free me to focus on the things I could change and release what I couldn't.

Developing a new relationship with my body gave me the power to deal with other things, too: personal issues in my life that I'd long been avoiding. They might have been scary, I realized, but they were not going to kill me. And I knew that if I addressed them, finally, I'd come out the other side a more authentic, better, happier person who was more in touch with herself. After that, doors started opening up. I began to really work on my marriage. It had not been going well, and I decided, "I'm not going to bullshit this anymore" (which was what I had been doing), but rather, that I was really going to commit to working on it, do the therapy, ask the hard questions, and have the difficult conversations. I did, and we did, and in the end we decided it made sense to move on.

All of those difficult, painful decisions had to happen. They came from asking myself: How do I really feel? This question alone had an incredible effect on my life. I started changing it up, having experiences that were more true to who I wanted to be, who I thought I was, and what I wanted in life. I was overcome with a thought: *Wow, this is way better.* I reinvestigated some of the Eastern practices that I'd been neglecting—meditation, yoga, and herbal remedies—and they helped me immensely with some of the symptoms such as sleep disturbances, low energy, mood swings, poor digestion, and weight changes that I experienced as I reacquainted myself with my passion for integrative medicine.

Those breakthroughs helped me in so many ways, including informing the way I now help women through menopause. Denying that it's happening or not giving this big event in your life its due never works. You will fail in your attempt to uncouple your body from your mind. It's an act of mental gymnastics that takes up too much energy in the end, and it isn't worth it. Let it go. One act—embracing menopause—will free up more compassion for yourself and allow you to offer your best self to the people around you.

Here's what I will tell you: no two of us is going to do this exactly the same way, and there isn't a cookie-cutter solution to any of our problems or quality-of-life issues. What I can offer is information that will give you a better understanding of what is happening and guide you through the solutions.

Only recently have complementary and alternative medicine started to become more accepted in mainstream medicine, partly because the research around the mind-body connection is irrefutable. I became a believer during my training. I was a chief resident at Cedars-Sinai when I met DD on the morning of her operation to remove large fibroid tumors in her uterus. For years, she'd tried to treat them holistically, but eventually surgery had become the only option. I'd come to her bedside in pre-op to answer any last-minute questions. DD had an unusual request: that I dab on some special essential oils that she'd brought with her "to bring clarity to the operating room." I looked at the small vial and then back at DD. Her look told me how important it was to her. "Okay," I said. "Sure, why not?" As I walked down the corridor to the OR, a thought landed on me with a thud: DD, a firm believer in alternative medicine, was placing her ultimate trust in a person she had just met and in a system that made her uneasy. It cost me nothing to entertain the request and show her the respect she deserved, even if I didn't understand it.

The surgery was very challenging. I remember it well even now. The next day, I went to check in on her. I can't tell you what a shock it was to see her hospital room. There was DD, propped up in bed, in a room festooned with Tibetan prayer flags and smelling of oils. Her friends who had redecorated had also brought in homemade soups for her to eat. DD's recovery was remarkable. She was up and out in record time.

Not long after, DD reached out and offered me a gift of meditation classes as a token of her gratitude. I declined, thinking that it seemed like a boundary violation. A year later, after I'd graduated, I found her phone number while cleaning out my desk and contacted her. It was a remarkable thing to see her outside the hospital. She was brimming with health and good cheer. She taught me Pilates and introduced me to the holistic and wellness communities of Los Angeles in the early 2000s. She taught me meditation and introduced me to Deepak Chopra and Ayurveda. She opened my eyes, heart, and mind to global healing traditions I'd had no idea about. What resulted was incredible: she deepened my capacity to listen and learn without judgment, as she had never judged my attachment to conventional or Western medicine. Instead, she nurtured my curiosity and desire to integrate the best of all possible worlds. Simply put, I would not be the doctor I am today had I not accepted her offer.

This book is not the culmination of all my learning. But I'm twenty-five years into this career, this life path, and I suspect that my desire to create this guide for you is that I've collected a critical mass of information. I want to share it with you in the hope that it will make your menopause transition more fulfilling—medically, physically, socially, and spiritually. I believe in my bones and hope with all my being that there's something in here that will connect with you. Let's get started.

PART I

What's Actually Going On?

The big changes have a biological basis. To understand why we are hotter than Oklahoma in August, it's helpful to understand our body's mechanics in a big-picture way.

When puberty rolled around, we were educated on that life change by some combination of a few sources of varying dependability: health class taught by the phys ed teacher, an awkward "the birds and the bees" talk with your folks, an eye-opening alternative "the birds and the bees" talk with an older sister, and the book *Are You There God? It's Me, Margaret* by Judy Blume. Tampons were intimidating. Someone told you not to swim in the ocean during your period because it attracted sharks. It was rough going. But it was still a celebrated passage. Hey, some kids hold period parties! (Look it up online. The cakes have a lot of red frosting.) Menopause deserves the same level of information, compassion, even celebration—which is to say, I would really like to score an invitation to your menopause soirée. But in the meantime, we really need to understand what the hell is going on with our changing bodies.

The problem is, as previously discussed, that not all doctors are well versed in menopause. There's no special training during medical school, and we get little to no specific education during our ob-gyn residency. (Instead, the lion's share of our time is spent learning about women's bodies during fertility, as our society is ageist and more than a smidge misogynistic—which is something we'll get to later.) If you're like many people who feel lacking in knowledge, consider this a health class exclusively for menopause. Bear with me, friends; there's need-to-know stuff in here. We'll go as quickly as possible. Let's start by defining some terms.

CHAPTER 1

The Basics

Premenopause: Before menopause. This is the span of time that started with your first period (menarche) and describes the time in life when a person is having a reliable menstrual cycle. These are the so-called childbearing years. People with uteruses are on a twenty-eight-day cycle, give or take a couple days. In this time, the hormones fluctuate in predictable patterns to ready the body for pregnancy; if the body detects none, it rids the uterus of the lining it had prepared. Fertility peaks in the midtwenties, but successful pregnancies—both natural and via fertility treatments—can occur well into the forties.

Perimenopause: This is a wobbly term that describes the time between premenopause and menopause. It often comes up in discussions about menopause, which is why we're addressing it here. But in fact, there's no consensus on what exactly "perimenopause" is. Plus, the very word makes some women squeamish. (Later on I'll make the case that we should banish it altogether.) *Peri* means "around," so technically this means "around menopause." During this span of time, the ratio of estrogen to progesterone levels starts to shift compared with where it was during your childbearing years. That hormonal change may manifest itself in how you feel. It can cause physical symptoms, such as hot flashes, and mental and emotional ones, such as mood changes or just feeling "off." Another sign, especially for people whose menstrual cycles have previously occurred with Swiss clock precision, is that their periods are thrown off. Patients of mine find this a disruptive time, particularly if they're used to a predictable cycle. They also report that premenstrual syndrome (PMS) symptoms can go pretty berserk, even if they hadn't experienced bad ones earlier in their lives. Breast tenderness can happen, so much so that women may think they're pregnant.

Okay, I have a radical idea: let's ban perimenopause. Hear me out. I want to share a phenomenon that happens weekly: A late-fortysomething patient comes into my office, saying she feels a little . . . off. Until recently, she bounced out of bed every morning after a solid seven hours of sleep, but now she tosses and turns all night and wakes up feeling groggy. Maybe her clothes are fitting more tightly than usual. Her emotions are all over the place, in ways that feel unfamiliar.

Sometimes she knows what I'm going to say and cringes in anticipation; other times, she has the look of someone who's just watched a puppy get run over by a Mack truck: *Sounds like you're in perimenopause*. In years past, that statement—"Sounds like you're in perimenopause"—provided huge relief and validation of a previously unacknowledged but very real change. More recently, I've noticed a shift. Some of us remain relieved that we are not crazy and that there is help. But others seem to feel accused of something, ashamed and pathologized.

The term *perimenopause* is, as I said before, wobbly. It doesn't really mean much. Women are still getting their periods, typically irregularly, perhaps with a change in the amount of bleeding. And they are experiencing symptoms that are common to menopause. But this could be because of the menopausal transition, or it could be something to do with fluctuating hormones, including stress hormones. It could happen when you're thirty-seven or forty-seven. All of these people are shuttled into the perimenopause category, but we don't have a definition of what it actually is. Definition-wise, the best I can say is that it's a stage in an ongoing physiological event. Doesn't clear things up, does it? The North American Menopause Society (NAMS) states, "As menopause approaches, cycles may vary by a week or more in one direction or another, but in general cycles move further apart—this marks a stage known as perimenopause." It's a safe, accurate definition, to be sure, but it still only skims the surface. Noticing shifting periods works only if you had predictable periods beforehand. And there are other reasons why periods may go off schedule. What if you don't have a uterus anymore and thus can't track your bleeding? So even that definition isn't particularly definitive.

If you're confused by the terminology, you're not alone—it is confusing. We've been throwing these words around for decades and to date have done a shitty job of explaining them. That would be okay—medicine is full of uncomfortable unknowns—if we didn't also load the thing up with all of this meaning. That's the part that pisses me off—because I say "perimenopause" and patients hear "beginning of the end." The airplane of youthfulness is starting its descent. Some women—a lot of women—have a really hard time with that. Honest to God, I'm not judging them. I've been there.

The reason that dealing with perimenopause is hard is individual. Some women are now faced with the reality that their window of fertility is closing. As a doctor, there are certain things I can fix and certain things I can't. I can't, for example, make your eggs more viable. And so, as the number of women who delay having a child grows, particularly among those with college and advanced degrees, the idea that there's always time to add to their family—it just isn't true forever, which can be a heavy realization. So they begin to feel as though, thanks to that one doctor's appointment, they're being forced to decide if they actually do want to have one more child, which has suddenly become a now-or-never proposition.

Some people are anxious about diseases associated with becoming older and the mammograms, colonoscopies, bone density scans, cardiac stress tests, and other surveillance measures to detect cancer, heart issues, and other age-related diseases. It's around this time that their friends start being diagnosed with diseases that up until now seemed to belong largely to their parents' generation. This can be hugely emotional, and when it comes up, I try to counter the fear with the empowerment that comes from being proactive and staying on top of surveillance plus focusing on lifestyle adjustments that can help stave off illness.

With that in mind, I want to introduce a phenomenon that we talk a lot about in medicine: inflammation. When you fall and sprain your ankle, which then swells up to twice its normal size, that's inflammation. It's part of the body's healing process—except not always. Menopause seems to trigger more chronic inflammation, and it manifests itself in ways that we can start to see. Psoriasis is a skin condition related to inflammation that worsens during menopause. Dry mouth and dry eyes are also linked with inflammation, as are certain orthopedic issues, such as frozen shoulder. So if, all of a sudden, you're noticing that these are happening to you, I am here to say: You're not crazy, and you're not alone!

In the time leading up to menopause, nearly 50 percent of women experience abnormal uterine bleeding, or AUB. It's an annoying disruption, but it can also have serious medical consequences, including anemia. Structural changes to the uterus, including fibroids, polyps, and adenomyosis (a condition similar to endometriosis), contribute to AUB, as do hormonal changes. But cancer of the cervix, uterus, fallopian tubes, or ovaries can be what is causing the abnormal bleeding. This is a massive topic in and of itself and outside the scope of this book, but if you are experiencing AUB, you should absolutely be evaluated by an experienced practitioner as soon as it happens in order to prevent or mitigate severe health ramifications.

I fully understand that I just said you have to look to the doctor "to prevent or mitigate severe health ramifications." I don't want to mince words, because the condition can be serious, but it is further evidence that there are biological and medical reasons for menopause-related anxiety. You should also know that if you happen to have a period that looks like a crime scene, don't panic; it's probably normal, but do go see your doc. If you haven't sensed it by now, this is how I speak to my patients: in objective, matter-of-fact terms, using data, best practices, and all of the other things in my doctor's tool kit. My hope is that if they arrive in a state of anxiety, they will leave reassured and calmer. That's not to say that every visit goes well and everything's copacetic. But that word *perimenopause*—what a trigger that one is. It's a doom-and-gloom-laden term that makes people feel crestfallen. It's the last stop before banishment to Dried-up Island. But the patients are literally thirty minutes older when they walk out of the appointment than when they came in. So why do they feel the sudden whiplash? Stupid perimenopause.

So screw it. Let's be done with it. I'm banning the term. From now on, you're premenopausal—in your childbearing years—or in menopause. If you're turning the book over to double-check that I'm an MD, I assure you that I am—which is how I can say with total confidence that not designating a patient as perimenopausal will not change the way I treat them. The guidelines around cancer screenings are based on age, and they change depending on whether you have a family history of a particular disease. If you come to me complaining of a dry vagina, we're going to treat your dry vagina, no matter if you're twenty-four or forty-four. And if having a child is your goal, we'll talk about that, too.

I should also say that I recognize that it's bullshit that we should conform our language to unreasonable social standards. I understand that the other tactic would be to reclaim the word. For what? It really serves little medical purpose. Anyway, it's far more worthwhile to focus our efforts on reclaiming menopause itself. Because if you do it right, it can be a lot of fun.

Menopause/postmenopause: These two terms are used interchangeably. It's when the menstrual cycle has ended, and, medically speaking, it denotes a different set of concerns doctors have about a woman's health. Menopause is what's called a retrospective determination. Once you've gone twelve consecutive months without a period, we know you have reached menopause.

But can we pause for a word on this word? Why do we hate the word *menopause*?

It can be problematic for a number of reasons, but I use the term so damn often that my own neutral response reflects my immersion in this work. Maybe that is not (yet) normal. I often hear that it sounds to many of you as though "men" are "pausing" or some other negative connotation. In fact, it is just the modern Latin term chosen (of course by male medical scientists) in the late nineteenth century to describe the time in a menstruating person's life when she ceases to menstruate. Period. The end. That is *all* it means. As far as its etymologic roots, that is . . .

The term *menopause* rose in popularity steeply from the 1960s until its peak in the last few years. When I was in medical school, the proper medical term was actually *climacteric*; there is even a prestigious medical journal bearing that name. Perhaps you prefer this word, which sounds amazing now that I say it again. It's the critical stage, juncture, decisive point! It's as if we should really be excited for the "big reveal." I use the term *menopause* in this book because it is most commonly understood. But you get to choose what you do with the information.

For women whose ovaries have been damaged or removed, that's called surgically induced menopause. For them, the changeover to menopause is immediate. If you have had a hysterectomy and don't have a visible manifestation of the menstrual cycle via bleeding (because, medically speaking, "the menstrual cycle" denotes all of the hormonally triggered changes), doctors will use a combination of your symptoms and experiences, and possibly blood tests, to determine when you've entered menopause.

I see you raising your hand out there. Can your doctor run a hormone test to determine whether you're in menopause? Most of the time, among women who are in their late forties or fifties, I wouldn't recommend it, for a few reasons. For starters, hormone levels go up and down continuously over the course of a twenty-eight-day cycle, so checking levels of certain hormones at one moment of time gives you hardly any usable information unless something is *way* off, indicating a different condition altogether. While you are still menstruating, no matter how irregularly, there's no telltale number that jumps out and says, "Just a heads-up, you're in menopause!" Also, regardless of where a woman finds herself on her trajectory, if she's experiencing menopause-like symptoms, we would still want to address them, even if her hormones appear to be "normal."

Here's the bottom line on how to determine when you're in the menopausal transition: When you come in to see me and say that your period is irregular, plus you've experienced hair loss and hot flashes and you want to kill your family, you've given me the diagnosis already. And if you've gone twelve consecutive months without a period, that is the textbook definition of menopause. It's like sending your eleven-year-old to the doctor because you are worried about the pubic hair, acne, and newfound brattiness that's shown up. You don't need a test to know that your kid's going through puberty. Now, if they had those symptoms at age five, that would be a different story. Same with menopause. If you're experiencing menopausal symptoms at age twenty-five, yes, we're going to do a hormone test. Because remember, menopause is not a disease. I'm going to say this once more because I cannot stress it enough: *If your doctor suggests you're going through menopause, he or she is not giving you a diagnosis. You're going through a normal part of life. And therefore there is no course of treatment for it.* But there are actionable steps you can take that will make your life better and easier. In the next section of the book, we'll break down all the symptoms, both familiar and lesser known, and relate them to the story we're telling about what's going on in your body.

It's okay if this all feels like a lot. When I look back at all I've told you, I feel the *whoosh* of a serious amount of information. There are a lot of people who are going through this with you. To prove it, I want to tell you about a few of them.

My Menopause Is Different from Your Menopause

No two women have the same menopause journey. And some are very different from the pack. I want to share the stories of some of my patients who agreed to appear in this book. You may see yourself in these stories, or you may learn about the experience of someone whose journey is very different.

Taking Control of Your Health Later in Life

MS is a sixty-five-year-old woman who went through a fairly smooth menopausal transition more than ten years ago but started seeing me only recently. A self-identified lesbian, she'd had negative experiences when going to the doctor earlier in her life, when physicians had lacked compassion and understanding. Because of this, she had rarely visited the gynecologist—at least not in the last decade. Her wife had insisted that she see me because of MS's family history of ovarian cancer and concerns about healthy aging. I admit, this is a scary one to have in your family tree. There are no effective screening protocols, so early detection is extremely difficult, and once it's in Stage 3 or 4, the mortality rate is 100 percent. It's the leading cause of death among all gynecological cancers, and it is a small comfort that the lifetime risk of developing it is less than 2 percent—though again, family history puts a different spin on things.

Together, MS and I created an overall health plan to address some of the health issues she was having at the moment, as well as plan for the future. They included lifestyle modifications, including exercise, sleep, stress reduction, dietary changes, and agreeing to annual visits with her primary care physician for prevention of other major medical conditions such as diabetes, hypertension, osteoporosis, and colon cancer. MS had never been pregnant (and therefore hadn't breastfed), which, medically speaking, put her at increased risk for some reproductive cancers, such as breast and ovarian. The appointment was an opportunity to address the barriers to care that women such as MS and many other LGBTQIA+ people experience and how those barriers harm people's health—and the fact that finding properly trained and understanding doctors can take the trauma out of a patient's experience. (For context, a survey by the Center for American Progress found that 8 percent of all LGBTQIA+ people had delayed or avoided seeking health care because of discrimination or disrespect by medical staff.) MS was given the opportunity to see a genetic counselor to learn whether she was one of the 10 percent of women who carry a known mutation that increases the risk of certain cancers. Our appointment was a long one, which was appropriate since MS was a new patient without much of a medical file to rely on, but in the end we created a plan for partnership and open communication. Now she sees me every year.

When Your Body Demands That You Get Heart Smart

At age forty-nine, AG suffered a myocardial infarction—a heart attack—which was the result of a spontaneous cardiac arterial dissection

(SCAD). It's an emergency condition in which a tear forms in an artery in the heart. AG didn't know she was having a heart attack, because heart attacks present differently in women from the way they do in men. She was experiencing neck pain, nausea, and fatigue, yet still made sure her family was off to face their day before calling for medical help. SCAD is a rare condition, and some studies suggest that 98 percent of people who experience it are women ages thirty to fifty, which indicates that it may be associated with hormones. Like many women with so-called microvascular heart disease or atypical heart disease, she was not a candidate for a stent because there was no blocked vessel. Instead, she was prescribed multiple medications and entered a cardiac rehabilitation program, which slowly and safely reintroduced her to day-to-day activities at home and caring for her family. Her entire life was thrown into chaos as she negotiated her new normal—including the acute sense of life's frailty engendered by her near-death experience.

By the time I saw AG, she was moving toward her menopausal transition and her periods had become increasingly heavy and painful. Her heavy bleeding was not only disrupting her daily life—soaking through pads, limiting her ability to go places, but she was a Pilates enthusiast and new grandmother with so much to look forward to! For other women experiencing heavy bleeding leading up to menopause, we'd entertain the use of hormones to get the situation under control, but with her cardiac history, that was a no-go. Anyway, she wasn't so hot on the idea of adding a new medication to her regimen. She preferred to depend on lifestyle changes and not prescriptions, probably because she was still grappling with what had happened to her not that long before and being thrust into a world of doctors' appointments, tests, scans, procedures, and more.

But the bleeding continued to the point that it was dangerous; in her case, it was creating what could be life-threatening anemia. As her blood counts drifted down, her heart was put under greater stress and

I was seriously concerned that she could suffer another heart attack as a result. Ultimately, we decided to place a progestin-containing IUD to counteract the estrogen dominance that was causing her bleeding. She later told me that she was gratified by its success and her ability to regain some control over her life. She knows that if she develops symptoms such as hot flashes, we can try herbs or acupuncture as long as her entire medical team approves.

Sometimes Menopause Comes Too Soon

KD and I first met when she was thirty-six years old. She was newly married—and newly diagnosed with Stage 3 breast cancer. What that meant was that her tumor was larger than 2 centimeters at the time of diagnosis—about the size of a shelled peanut. Tests also revealed more than twenty cancer-involved lymph nodes. That meant that the cancer had spread into the immune system and potentially was already widely distributed throughout her body. Owing to her young age and how much of her lymph system was involved, she was given a full battery of treatment, including surgery, chemotherapy, and radiation. I'll never forget the first day we met; KD wore a cute scarf wrapped around her bald head and told me she was scared that she'd never have the family she dreamt of. And the chemotherapy-induced menopause she was experiencing brought with it a whole host of issues: near-constant hot flashes, almost no libido, and painful sex due to vaginal dryness. Her doctors had let her know that her period might never return. Although some young women facing chemo-induced menopause are offered the opportunity to retrieve eggs for fertility sparing prior to treatment, that option wasn't open to her. (Egg retrieval involves the use of hormones to accelerate ovulation, which might have had the effect of accelerating the cancer as well, which was why it wasn't an option for her.) With the support of her world-renowned oncologist and after doing a thorough literature review to determine what would be safe and effective, we implemented a plan to bring her comfort and restore her sense of self. Vaginally administered topical estradiol—which is a synthetic but biologically identical hormone that stands in for estrogen—is known to remain largely in the vaginal tissue, rather than circulating in the body, and helps to replenish blood flow, moisture, and lubrication and increase sexual response. And since topical estradiol isn't absorbed into the bloodstream enough to create clinically significant issues, the potential for it to "feed" her cancer did not exist. Then we started looking at other nonhormonal ways to give her a better quality of life, including using herbs or botanical medicines such as black cohosh to safely quell her hot flashes. KD also started working closely with a local doctor of Chinese medicine and undergoing acupuncture to ameliorate some of her chemotherapy-induced side effects, as well as those classic to menopause, such as anxiety, joint pain, and difficulty sleeping. She defied the odds, her periods returned, and her oncologist cleared her for pregnancy. She continued utilizing traditional Chinese medicine and conceived two children three years apart. I had the honor of delivering both of her babies. Now she's in the midst of fine-tuning her supplements and lifestyle as she transitions to menopause. She remains cancer free fifteen years after our first meeting.

CHAPTER 2

Hormones and "The Big Four"

Clinically speaking, when your period doesn't show up for twelve consecutive months, you're in menopause. So what happens if you're on contraception that reduces the frequency of your period or eliminates it entirely? Is it harder to determine when your cycle is off if you didn't have one to begin with? Yes, but it just means that, as physicians, we have to look for other clues to determine whether you're in menopause: things such as sleeping patterns changing, newly developed sexual complaints (dry vagina and reduced libido, for example), hot flashes, hair loss, and mood changes. If you are still using hormonal contraception at age fifty, I would suggest asking your doctor about discontinuing it. I'll be up front with you and say that this is a somewhat controversial take. So I want to share my thoughts.

If you're taking hormonal contraception for pregnancy prevention,

I totally get it. I wouldn't want a late-in-life surprise pregnancy, either. In that case, you may want to consider an alternative, such as an IUD. However, a lot of women remain on hormonal contraception for the symptom management aspect. Maybe you're on it to control painful periods, PMS symptoms, depression, or endometriosis. For these patients, I usually initiate a conversation about switching over to menopausal hormone therapy. This uses different hormones and in different doses to achieve some of the same symptom management goals, as well as address some physical changes that happen during menopause. There's more here to dive into, but the CliffsNotes version is: There's reason to believe that the hormone progestin used in standard low-dose birth control may carry a small, but not insignificant, increased breast cancer risk. Many women do decide that it's worth the risk, and it's their choice, completely. But if your fertility has dropped significantly (and if you're in menopause, it definitely has), there are other options in the form of menopausal hormone therapy that can provide symptomatic relief that may be safer for you in the long run. If you bring this up with your doctor, don't be surprised if you're met with an attitude of "If it's not broken, don't fix it." Press your physician on their reasoning, on why they don't want to make a change. And if you feel as though you're not getting a satisfactory answer, seek out a second opinion.

To get just a little more into the weeds: It's not uncommon for practicing doctors to disagree with standards of practice. What I mean is that sometimes, one of the big groups that represent doctors, such as the American Medical Association or the American College of Obstetricians and Gynecologists, comes out with new guidelines for something, such as the age when people should have their first mammogram. The Food and Drug Administration also sets safety standards and oversees drug approvals and usages. One of the disagreements my personal medical practice has with the FDA guidelines has to do with MHT: it allows for MHT that contains the hormone progestin. I avoid progestin, if possible. The reason is that I don't see why I'd use progestin, with its acknowledged risks, when micronized progesterone—biologically identical to what our own bodies make—is available. The reality is that the data on progesterone are not as abundant as those on progestin, but it does appear to be safer, especially regarding breast cancer risk.

I know that those three words—menopausal hormone therapy (MHT and what used to be called hormone replacement therapy, or HRT)—are themselves very controversial. That controversy may be why your doctor is opposed to switching your prescription. MHT has been maligned owing to years of subpar science and a lack of compassion for women experiencing menopause symptoms, who are expected to endure the body changes, mood swings, depression, and other aspects that menopausal people experience.

Before we go on, I have a thought. It occurs to me that we should have a quick chat about hormones, what they are and how they work. It'll be quick, I promise.

The Chemical Messengers Running the Show

We talk a lot about hormones, but it occurs to me that unless you went to med school, you may not know exactly what they are. I think one reason doctors shy away from explaining it to their patients is because it's such a delightfully complicated and fraught conversation! But you're here to learn, so here we go.

Simply put, hormones are chemical messengers. This is one way your body talks to itself, and it's not only the ovaries and uterus but also the pancreas and gut, even your fat, skin, muscles, bones, and heart that communicate with one another via hormone signaling. The time of day these chemicals are released and in what quantity are a big part of why our bodies function the way they do. For instance, if you've ever popped a melatonin pill at the end of a cross-country flight to adjust to the new time zone and get some shut-eye, you've taken a supplement of the hormone that signals the body that it's time to go to sleep. The body's hormonal pathway is called the *endocrine system*. It's one of numerous ways that the brain talks to the body, the other being the nervous system, which controls movement and bodily responses to things such as heat and pain. Hormones are responsible for a boggling number of human functions: energy level, stress, metabolism, immune response, growth, and, of course, reproduction. Evolutionarily speaking, they are fine tuned to keep us alive as a species. In ancient times, if you were a hunter-gatherer in the bush and caught sight of a tiger, you'd get a rush of adrenaline that would give your body the extra oomph to run fast and far to avoid being the tiger's lunch. The hormones that control falling asleep and waking up are linked to sunrise and sunset. I'm not sure if being "hangry" is an evolutionary adaptation, but that state of ravenous rage is absolutely the result of hormones.

The hormones we are focusing on here fall into a category called steroid sex hormones. I'm going to focus on the Big Four: estrogen, progesterone, testosterone, and dehydroepiandrosterone (DHEA).

Estrogen is responsible for physical feature changes at puberty such as breast development and pubic hair growth. It is also required for building up the lining of the uterus and shedding it through menstruation. It also impacts cholesterol control and bone growth and affects the brain, skin, and heart. The ovaries—and specifically the eggs—are responsible for our supply of estrogen. The forms it takes vary throughout our cycle and lifetime. Estradiol (E2) is what most of us know as "estrogen"; this dominates reproduction and menstruation. Estriol (E3) increases during pregnancy; estrone (E1) dominates after menopause, when the ovarian supplies of E2 and E3 have diminished or disappeared. There are differences in the way our body's tissue responds to these various forms.

The presence or absence of estrogen carries implications for the development of cancer, osteoporosis, neurodegenerative diseases, cardiovascular issues, gynecological problems such as endometriosis, and obesity, and the intricate interactions among multiple hormones, including estrogen, can have a significant impact on mood, sex drive, and weight maintenance.

Progesterone is a magical steroid sex hormone that is produced by a temporary structure in your ovary called the corpus luteum. I am fascinated by this; the ovary, itself an organ, develops the corpus luteum under the influence of multiple hormones in a complex feedback loop with the brain that is meant to facilitate a once-a-month egg release event that lasts a mere twelve to twenty-four hours. The corpus luteum then literally implodes and disappears. When we experience a menstrual cycle, the ovary chooses *one* egg out of the one million we are born with to release during ovulation in order to make pregnancy possible. This process happens three to four hundred times over a person's lifetime. The corpus luteum produces progesterone to support an early conception by creating a fluffy uterine lining and prohibiting uterine muscle spasms. If we don't get pregnant, the corpus luteum disintegrates and our progesterone level declines until the next cycle. In this way, progesterone keeps the estrogen level in check over the course of many decades. Over time, their close relationship to one another transforms. As we stop ovulating on a regular basis in our middle years, not only does our estrogen level decline, but progesterone's modulation of estrogen's stimulating influence also declines. For instance, estrogen grows the lining of the uterus, but with less progesterone around, the lining can more aggressively stimulate and overgrow, resulting in increased bleeding and a risk of developing precancerous or cancerous growths. Additionally, the shift in balance may result in less of the emotional feeling of softness and relaxation associated with progesterone's effect. Increases in irritability and anxiety in the premenstrual part of the cycle can result. I like to see estrogen as the more dominant, aggressive hormone and progesterone as her containing, harmonizing sister.

Testosterone is an androgen, which means that it's involved in the development of masculine traits and reproduction. Although we may think of it as a "male" hormone, women actually have more testosterone than estradiol in their younger years. Produced in the ovaries and adrenal glands located at the top of the kidneys, testosterone interacts with other hormones to help create strong bones, lean body mass (muscles), and metabolism and to some extent influences libido. Hair, skin, and vaginal mucosa are also affected by testosterone, the level of which also declines with age.

DHEA, or dehydroepiandrosterone, is also produced primarily in the adrenals—and to a much lesser extent in the ovaries. This is what is known as a *precursor hormone*. That means it has the ability to "morph" into different hormones, depending on what the body needs—either estradiol (a form of estrogen) or testosterone; to do so, it requires enzymes (special proteins that set off chemical reactions) that convert one substance into another. DHEA is the body's most abundant steroid hormone, and it's made from cholesterol.

Let's Not Forget the Thyroid

Thyroid hormones have an intimate relationship with sex hormones. Women have more thyroid issues than men do, and there is often an uptick in problems around the time of menopause. Many menopausal symptoms mimic those of an irregular thyroid, including weight gain, mood issues, skin and hair changes, and menstrual irregularity. Since those symptoms can result from either menopause or thyroid issues (or both), they can be difficult to differentiate. How often do I have a patient who hopes that all of her woes could be fixed by addressing her thyroid? (Me. I'm in that camp.) It turns out that estrogens do influence thyroid function to some extent through something called *subclinical hypothyroidism*, which occurs in about 15 percent of women over age sixty and up to about 10 percent of midlife adults. If your doctor suspects that a thyroid malfunction may be in play, he might order a blood test and prescribe medicine to replace the missing thyroid hormones.

So let's bring the discussion back to menopause. The reason that menopause happens in the first place is that estrogen production in the ovaries peters out, which happens because of the natural, age-related loss of eggs over time. And when estrogen declines, so does progesterone. During this fairly massive hormonal shift is when people experience the strongest physical and emotional symptoms. The body likes homeostasis, meaning that it prefers when things stay the same. This shift, however hard it is to define, is going on during the transition, so although you may be getting periods, you may be skipping months and your bleeding and/or cramping could be getting worse, plus you're feeling the aftershocks of your body's constantly adjusting to the declining levels of hormones. When the hormone levels stabilize, the symptoms often resolve, too.

My Best Friend Said I Should Get My Hormones Checked . . . and Other Unscientific Advice

When a patient comes in and tells me that their therapist/nutritionist/trainer/girlfriend told them to get their hormone levels checked, I face-palm mentally every time. Usually they're looking for some secrets baked into the numbers that would tell them what to eat or to avoid, whether it's better for them to work out in the morning or at night, that they can improve their productivity by orienting their workspace to the east, or some other fad that uses pseudoscience to provide an air of precision medicine.

There are a few reasons I would check a patient's hormone levels, as they provide specific answers *to a medical doctor*. For instance, if you are in your twenties or thirties and are exhibiting menopausal symptoms, that might indicate that your ovaries aren't producing enough estrogen and we have a problem on our hands. Or if you've had a hysterectomy but still have ovaries (and thus don't have a period to track), we'd do blood work to look at some markers. Let's say you got the hormone test anyway and it indicates that your estrogen levels are fine, but you're still feeling the symptoms of menopause: bad sleep, vaginal dryness, hot flashes. I wouldn't send you packing just because the test came back without a clear menopause diagnosis. I'd treat your symptoms just the same!

Here are a few reasons I'm telling you all of this.

◆ We don't really have adequate reference ranges or an understanding of what amounts to "normal" for each hormone. It's not like blood sugar or cholesterol levels, where we have a good understanding of what's healthy versus what's dangerous. This is actually a huge area of research at the moment. If you're interested in this work, I'd direct you to Sara E. Hill, PhD, a psychologist and the author of the book *This is Your Brain on Birth Control: The Surprising Science of Women, Hormones, and the Law of Unintended Consequences.* She is working to devise ways for women to better understand their personal hormonal changes throughout their menstrual cycle and be able to map them against how they are feeling both physically and emotionally. This is a fascinating extension of so-called precision medicine, in which treatments and interventions are crafted specifically to the cellular needs of the person taking them. Incidentally, venture capitalism is also really interested in this area of science. On the other hand, the fact that we don't have more *academic* research into this area says a lot about how much effort research medicine has been willing to invest to understand women's bodies, with their ever-fluctuating hormones.

◆ If you come to me and say you are having an array of symptoms such as hot flashes, skin and hair issues, or sex drive changes, simply doing a one-off hormone test can reveal a little bit of information but will seldom tell you definitively what's going on. I know I've said this already, but it bears repeating: a single blood test will give you the hormone ratios in a moment in time, but your hormone levels are constantly changing and are influenced by a number of bodily systems, both major and minor. The numbers you get one day won't be the same the next.

◆ For people who have taken medications or supplements that change their hormone levels, such as birth control, cancer treatment, or gender confirmation therapy, it adds another level of complexity to your menopause journey.

◆ If you're in the eighth circle of menopause hell and worry that what you're experiencing is now your lot in life, don't be discouraged. Your menopausal symptoms will improve, and there are plenty of ways we can help make things better, both when you're in the thick of the change and afterward, when you're adjusting to your new body. (Parts II, III, and IV of this book are devoted to this!)

◆ In my practice, I have patients who tell me they want to try a certain treatment because their friend had such a great response to it, and then a few weeks later, they come in disheartened because it didn't work for them. The complexity of hormones—and the fact that everyone's body chemistry is unique—is why different people have such different outcomes. Or why, for you, a certain treatment had side effects or unintended consequences. The thing that works for one person may have a very different effect on someone else. As an aside: if a doctor is telling you with 100 percent certainty that a certain hormone treatment is going to fix everything that's wrong with you, go find another doctor. There's no way that doc could possibly know this. The brightest and most concerned doctors are up front about the complexity of hormone treatment and offer to be a partner with you as you try out treatment and keep an open mind moving forward.

◆ Last, I want to offer a brief "buyer beware." Many of my colleagues and I have been shocked by the number of doctors who seem to have predatory practices. They capitalize on their patients' vulnerabilities around the time of menopause, and to many of us, it seems as though they are using the emotional strife of some of their patients as a moneymaking opportunity. So if you are being offered an array of fancy-sounding and very expensive tests (which are not usually covered by insurance) and an even more dizzying array of treatments, take a long, hard look at why. Are your symptoms dire enough to warrant all-out warfare? Meaning if you're experiencing some hot flashes, some mood changes, some vulvar discomfort—which is highly unpleasant but not insurmountable—have you exhausted more simple, over-the-counter solutions before going to a Cadillac treatment that'll be cost and time intensive? I'm not trying to devalue your experience or symptoms. Hormones are crazy, and their changes manifest themselves in equally crazy ways. But our response to these manifestations doesn't have to be.

Let's put this into practice, because I know it can be hard for people to question their doctors. After all, that white coat is a signal of omniscience! Except . . . that's not always the case. If your doctor wants to test your hormones, here are the most important things to ask them:

◆ What are you trying to learn from this test?
◆ What number would constitute a "normal" result versus an abnormal result? And if the test comes back with an abnormal result, what would you do in response? What kind of treatment would be in play?
◆ What scientific evidence or reasoning are you using to interpret results and recommend a treatment plan?
◆ How much will this cost? If there's a suggested treatment, how much would that cost?

How Does Cancer Change Things?

Certain cancers—particularly breast and gynecological cancers—have a hormonal aspect: they can use sex hormones for fuel, similarly to the way that testosterone can play a role in prostate cancer among men. And since a drop-off in hormones is at the heart of menopause, it stands to reason that cancer will change a person's menopause trajectory.

For those who are in treatment for cancer or who are, like me, in remission, there are some important distinctions that I'll call out throughout the book. Here are a few things to know from the outset: The timeline of menopause is completely different if you have had surgery to remove your ovaries, called an oophorectomy. If a patient has a bilateral oophorectomy, meaning that both ovaries are removed, she will go into menopause immediately. If she has a unilateral oophorectomy, she can still get periods, though it's likely that she'll experience menopause earlier. And if a person has a hormone-receptive tumor, she may take medications that further suppress her estrogen production, which could make menopausal symptoms worse.

So yes, on top of cancer, you get a whole new round of hot flashes and mood swings. It can all be really overwhelming. And although there are some menopause-related treatments that'll be off limits to people who are dealing with cancer or remission, this book is full of many recommendations that are absolutely kosher for you—and may help with some of the lasting effects of cancer, too.

A question I am asked a lot is what happens if a woman has a "partial hysterectomy." This isn't really a medical term, but it's used by patients to describe removing the uterus without removing the ovaries. These people will not go into surgically induced menopause, but the data do suggest that they will go into menopause at a younger age. Without a period to track, it's harder to know when they are in their menopausal transition. And for those who've undergone chemotherapy, in some cases it sets them up for early menopause as well. It seems that certain drugs can cause premature ovarian insufficiency, or POI, meaning that the ovaries stop producing estrogen earlier in a woman's life. Up to 50 percent of childhood cancer survivors have POI. Temporary or permanent chemotherapy-induced POI affects between a quarter and 100 percent of breast cancer survivors.

What this all adds up to is that, yes, cancer can change what your menopause trajectory looks like. Big cancer centers and academic institutions often have resources, such as specially trained experts, as well as support groups, that can help you navigate the physical and emotional changes.

I'm Here to Tell You: You Don't Know How You'll Deal with Cancer Until You Have to Deal with Cancer

It was near the beginning of my menopausal journey that I was diagnosed with breast cancer. I was forty-seven. Being a women's health doctor with an interest in the more challenging medical aspects of the specialty—and having had a close relationship with our local breast cancer experts—I had developed into something of a niche specialist in the gynecologic care of those with premenopausal breast cancer. So when I got the diagnosis, I was fortunate to have that all-star network of specialists and access to the latest resources and information. Since I have the opportunity here, I'll give a shout-out to my all-women team of doctors: oncologist Dr. Philomena McAndrew, breast surgeon Dr. Kristi Funk, and radiation oncologist Dr. May Lin Tao.

So the medical part was taken care of. But what I didn't know was how I'd be as a patient. In the United States, about one in eight women develops breast cancer, and in my practice I'd seen all sorts of expressions of that experience. There were those who were vocal about their diagnosis and kept their friends, family, and social media apprised of their treatments. At the other end of the spectrum, some kept it hush-hush from all but their inner circle, sometimes even just a partner. For as out loud as I think I live my life, I tended to the latter group. But it wasn't to keep up some sort of professional facade or because I thought I could handle it on my own. I really rejected the vulnerability. I was initially quite secretive about my diagnosis, mostly because I did not want to hear about anyone else's feelings regarding my condition. Does that make me sound callous? I hope not. If you've ever been through a big, difficult life event—think divorce, a family member struggling with addiction, job loss—you'll know that a lot of the feedback and "sympathy" you get is about how your experience makes other people feel. They relate it to their life. They utilize insufficient comparisons. Sometimes you end up consoling them because they're upset about what's happening to you! It's a little mind bending, and when I was in the thick of it, I didn't have the bandwidth to invite too many people into my goings-on.

Eventually, I found my way into an incredible, informal group of survivors who call themselves "The Girls" (wink wink, nudge nudge), where I left my cocoon of detachment and learned to accept support. I also learned quite a few facts that I hadn't even learned from my medical team, such as reviews of specific medicines and how to deal with various side effects. We meet in person or online every month and share long, funny, poignant, and informative email threads every day. Truly lifesaving stuff.

* * *

No one is going to care more about your health than you. By absorbing all of this information you will be empowered to have informed conversations with your doctors, enabling you to process what they're telling you and have a role in the decision-making process. This background knowledge—especially about hormones—will give you necessary knowledge as we roll into part II, learning about the symptoms of menopause, as well as how to find relief and improve the aging trajectory.

I hear some of the older women who attend my Menopause Bootcamps tell the younger ones, "You're lucky if you reach menopause." It sounds a little glib at first and tone-deaf if you're the one drenched in your sweat-wicking shirt and wondering when your hair will stop falling out. But deep down, we know it's true. We get to age, and there's privilege in that. It's a great time for us, as well!

We're not very far into the book, and I'm sure you've already sensed my frustration with the medical establishment. We have let down women, nonbinary and trans people, really anybody who doesn't fit the traditional gender construct. But that's starting to change, albeit slowly. For instance, we know that estrogen almost certainly has a large role in brain function. Two-thirds of people who are diagnosed with Alzheimer's disease are women. Shocking, right? And researchers such as Lisa Mosconi, the director of the Women's Brain Initiative and associate director of the Alzheimer's Prevention Clinic at Weill Cornell Medical College/NewYork-Presbyterian Hospital in New York City, along with her colleague Roberta Diaz Brinton, the director of the UA Center for Innovation in Brain Science at the University of Arizona Health Sciences, are trying to figure out what they call the "menopause connection." It seems that the sudden loss of estrogen triggers changes in the brain, including a fall in glucose metabolism that causes the brain to use ketone bodies—in particular the myelin sheaths that protect neurons—as a supplemental fuel source. Understanding this relationship will almost certainly open new avenues for prevention and treatment.

Still, science has more to uncover. And since we seem to be going through a Menopause Renaissance (even Hollywood is getting on board), we can, I hope, look forward to greater understanding of menopausal people's bodies and more innovations in how we can give them relief and better health.

Laid out like this, menopause sounds like a slow-moving train with us tied to the tracks. Yes, menopause presents challenges. Sometimes it downright sucks. But I'll say it again: there are things you can do to make this transition less uncomfortable—that's why you're here. And *Menopause Bootcamp* is here for you. You are not alone.

Worksheet:
What Should I Ask Myself Before Seeing My Doctor?

You're now flush with new knowledge about the biological gears at work. Next we're going to talk about how this relates to *your* experiences. There are some questions that are helpful to ask yourself—and they just so happen to be the questions that your doctor should be asking to ensure that you get the help you deserve during your transition. The answers to these questions will also help you clarify your goals, which are almost always related to your quality of life. Be your own sleuth, write down your findings, and the next time you have a gynecologist or general practitioner appointment, bring them with you. Here are a few questions to start:

QUESTION	ANSWER
Has your sex life changed? Is sex or masturbation painful? Have you noticed changes in your libido?	
How have you been sleeping? Approximately how many hours a night of shut-eye do you get? If you're not a great sleeper, do you have problems falling asleep, or do you find yourself getting up throughout the night?	
Have you noticed an increased need to urinate, either during the day or while you're in bed? Do you leak or lose urine during activities?	
Think about where you're at emotionally. Have you noticed a change in your mood? If so, is it like PMS, where you are a little all over the place for a few days at a time, or do you kind of want to kill the people you love on a fairly consistent basis? (That was my experience at least.)	

QUESTION	YOUR ANSWER
How often do you have hot flashes, and how manageable are they? Are you able to let them pass, or are they starting to affect your day-to-day life? Are they predictable, meaning that you know you'll hot flash before bed, for example, or in the lead-up to a stressful event like a big presentation?	
Do you have a support system? Are there people in your life whom you talk to about the issues going on in your life? Would you find more emotional support helpful?	

PART II

So How Are You Doing?

The medical side of menopause can feel like a whole new world. Let's explore it.

Timing: good for comedians, bad for menopause. It's something I hear from my patients and have experienced myself. Picture it: You're in your mid- to late-forties. You're the most self-accepting about your life that you've ever been, because you've made a lot of the big choices having to do with career, marriage, family, living situation. If you have kids, they're out of diapers and may be on their way out of the nest. In your relationships—with friends, family, perhaps a partner, and also yourself—you feel you can be honest. And that other big relationship—the one you have with your body—is more peaceful than it was in your teens and twenties and probably your thirties as well. Maybe what I'm describing doesn't speak exactly to you. Certainly everyone has a different journey, different successes and hardships. But it's nearly universal among the people whom I meet and speak with that the forties are when you finally feel as though you know yourself.

And then one day you wake up and your sheets are soaked. Or you're on a train and suddenly the temperature in the car goes to 95 degrees and it's imperative that you take off as many clothes as is socially acceptable.

Welcome to Hot Flash City.

Shit. Not only do hot flashes suck and seem to come on at just the wrong time—right before a presentation, as you're walking into a cocktail party, in the midst of a tête-à-tête with your person—it's also one of the symptoms that reminds you that the body that you've grown to understand and respect and even love is changing in fundamental and unpredictable ways. The symptoms themselves are a pain to deal with. But emotionally they can also be extremely disorienting. That's what a lot of women say is the real struggle of menopause, not feeling like themselves anymore. As in *Invasion of the Body Snatchers*, where you become a person you don't recognize. Or you become your mother.

As I said: *Shit.*

As a doctor, one of the ways I can support you is by helping to treat your symptoms as they arise. That's why I went through all of the biological changes going on in part I. I think it's empowering to know why, biologically, you're experiencing these symptoms; it helps you make more informed decisions as you decide whether and how to respond to your body's changes.

Are We Having *Symptoms*, or Are We Having *Experiences*?

Words are really important, and so I want to have a discussion about the word *symptom*. We have already established that menopause, like puberty, is not a disease and should not be treated as such. So why am I using the word *symptom* when I've already said that it isn't a pathology or disease?

First, I am a doctor, and we use the term *symptom* as a descriptor. I know that "symptom" is already a negatively weighted word, and I think, from a medical perspective, that my patients dislike the changes that are happening to them. Hot flashes, incontinence, muscle injuries—none of them is so great. And it's the language that health care providers use among one another. So I think it's helpful to give you insights into this language so you can be an even more active participant in your own care.

This is another way in which medicine and insurance create a toxic confluence. As a physician who considers herself progressive, I try to work to change the system, while remaining a die-hard advocate for my patients.

At the end of chapter 3, you'll have an opportunity to complete a worksheet that you and your doctor can use to make a game plan to treat your symptoms. If this ever feels like a lot, please keep in mind that there are a lot of ways to help and there's no one-size-fits-all solution. It takes a little work, but it'll be worth it.

* * *

A note about Ayurveda . . .

I've told you a few times now about my training in Ayurveda and that it plays a role in the kind of doctor that I am today. Now I want to tell you why.

First, I want to tell you about holism. It's a way of seeing the world—nature and humanity—as being fundamentally interconnected. It can also apply to our bodies. All of the systems of the body are interwoven—and not just the organs and muscles and skin but the physical body, mind, and spirit. Take a moment to consider the beautiful complexity of it all. We are all made up of systems that are both influenced by and emit influence to the world outside ourselves. We are part of the larger whole.

Holism is at the heart of Ayurveda, which is loosely translated as "the science of life." It began in the Indian subcontinent between four thousand and five thousand years ago, and its development paralleled the rise of traditional Chinese medicine.

Because each of us is a system of systems that's part of a larger system, things function the best when we are all in balance. In Ayurveda, we talk about illness as being a state of imbalance, so we want to prevent imbalance from happening and restore balance when it does. It's done through daily routines and lifestyle, diet, body therapies, yoga and meditation, breath work, and the use of botanical medicines and herbs. We are in balance when we work with nature, which also means eating locally and seasonally and operating with a respect for the balances that exist in nature.

I want to give you a little terminology. *Pancha maha bhutas* are, in Ayurveda, the building blocks of life: ether, air, water, fire, and earth. Each of these has its own characteristics: hot or cold, dry or moist, heavy or light, stable or mobile. And individuals have their own mix of all these building blocks and the ways they manifest themselves in the body.

If you're a little perplexed, I completely understand. You're reading a medical book by a medical doctor, and here I am talking about *pancha maha bhutas*. But if you dive into the Ayurvedic texts, you'll find that they are uncannily perceptive about how the human body works. They just use terminology that is unfamiliar. For instance, the texts offer detailed and scientifically accurate depictions of cardiovascular, lymphatic, immune, central and peripheral nervous, musculoskeletal, and digestive systems, as well as the reproductive tract. Ayurveda uses much different terminology than Western medicine does, and inherent to it is the interconnectedness of these systems.

When a person is sick, an Ayurvedic practitioner would search for the imbalance. Since they are trained to see the interwovenness of the body and the world, they think expansively about what could be causing a patient discomfort or disease. Let's take an easy example. A person goes to a doctor—any doctor, of Ayurvedic or Western persuasion—and says that they are suffering from horrible headaches. That practitioner then finds out that they just started a new job and are working overnights, their sleep has been horrible, and their body clock has gone haywire. An Ayurvedic doctor would say that the patient has an alteration of their *dosha*, or constitution. The Western doctor would say that their circadian rhythm is disrupted and the disruption is manifesting itself neurologically.

Both of the practitioners arrived at the same conclusion based on the same information. The Western doctor looked for a problem; the Ayurvedic doctor looked for an imbalance. But one of the things I like about the Ayurvedic approach is that if I were approaching a diagnosis, I would look for other imbalances. Is the new job stressful, and what impact is that having on the person's mental well-being? How is the new job affecting the patient's ability to socialize with friends and loved ones or their relationship—and is it causing them spiritual distress?

What Ayurvedic practitioners see as remedies also differ from those of Western doctors. For example, food and lifestyle are seen as enormous influences that need to be understood for the body to be in harmony. Breath, or prana, is an essential element of our life force. Ayurvedic practitioners also use essential oils, herbs, roots, plants, and spices for their medicinal qualities. One big difference between these treatments and the kinds of prescriptions that are filled at the pharmacy is that (1) they are often used preventively, before a small imbalance leads to a problematic big imbalance, and (2) it takes longer for them to work, and they need to be taken consistently.

Pretty much forever, there has been a loud group of Western doctors who have zero use for this way of thinking. I don't want to get into the reasons why, because the reasons are classist, date back to our colonial histories of conquering, denigrating, and erasing indigenous practices, and all around bum me out. Instead, I want to talk about what those old-fashioned, close-minded doctors are missing. Ayurveda helps us see the patient as a whole. It increases options for helping them because we are open minded in looking for causes of discomfort or issues in unexpected ways. And many of the solutions—lifestyle changes, herbal supplements—don't come with the kinds of side effects that need to be controlled as so often happens in Western medicine.

Ironically, in the last couple decades, major US institutions have been widening their thinking. Sometimes they're going back to traditional texts and subjecting them to academic medical rigor. And they're confirming the value of so many traditional practices and treatments through research. You've probably heard, for example, how many scientists are interested in microbiome research, how the mouth microbiome has connections to the cardiac system and the gut microbiome influences the brain.

It's a disservice to millions of Ayurvedic practitioners who have helped people for thousands of years to finally recognize their work only when contemporary Western doctors recognize its value. Disservice isn't even the right word. It's insulting.

To be clear, I'm not saying that one is better than the other. My medical worldview is seen through the lens of both. It helps me diagnose acute problems and lay out solutions for the patient, while also seeing the larger picture. It connects me to my practice. I use Ayurveda in my own life to give me a deeper understanding of where I fit into the world, which helps me relate to patients.

Ayurveda and traditional Chinese medicine are referred to as "complementary medicine," which I find to be pejorative. It treats them as second-class citizens to the dominant Western outlook. I think that Ayurveda enhances my Western understanding, and it provides answers when my traditional medical training seems to fall short.

I've been training in Ayurveda for years, and I am still a student. But what I'm hoping you take away from this is: You are more than your symptoms. You are an entire person, who is a universe unto yourself. A compassionate doctor will see you like that, too.

CHAPTER 3

The Symptoms of Menopause

I think the most straightforward way to give you all of this information is to go symptom by symptom, going from most to least common. A ton of them relate to fluctuating hormone levels, some of them relate to aging, and for others we don't quite know the mechanisms. This is the section where we deal with the body, and after that we're going to deal with the mind. I'm going to address this stuff clinically because I think it's important that you have the information you need, which will give you an even deeper understanding of some of this than your doctor does if they're not doing extracurricular training in menopause. You don't have to read this in order. Find the symptoms that speak to you.

> ## Hot Flashes and Menopausal Hormone Therapy:
> ## Can Someone Please Turn Up the AC?

If you play a word association game with "menopause," the first thing most people will say is "hot flashes." It's among the top three most common symptoms during the transition—about 75 to 80 percent of women experience them. You may not be sleeping that great, but you can explain it away by saying that you've got a lot on your mind. And yeah, you're more irritable, but you're trying to keep a lot of plates in the air! Hot flashes constitute the *aha!* moment. So pour yourself a big glass of ice-cold water (yup, it actually works) and let's dig in.

The Cause of Hot Flashes

Doctors aren't totally sure what causes hot flashes, but it seems that the body's thermometer stops working properly. The body is going through two things at once: a slight increase in core body temperature and a lowered thermoneutral zone, meaning that our ability to maintain the core body temperature required for cellular functions has changed. For example, when you're out in the world and your body adjusts seamlessly from being outside in the snow to being inside, where there's a big fire in the fireplace, it's a sign that it has a wide and functioning thermoneutral zone. We want to live in the sweet spot between shivering and sweating, but during menopause, that window narrows. That thermoneutral zone change is attributed to menopause's estrogen drop, but there are at least three other hormones that seem to play a role: gonadotrophin, luteinizing hormone, and norepinephrine. (I wasn't kidding when I said that hormones are incredibly complicated, and there's no such thing as isolating one; they are always working in concert together.)

What Hot Flashes Feel Like

According to Dr. Robert Freedman at Wayne State University School of Medicine, a hot flash is "a rapid and exaggerated heat dissipation response, consisting of profuse sweating, peripheral vasodilation, and feelings of intense, internal heat." In other words: holy Scottsdale in August, it's hot in here! For most people, hot flashes last from one to five minutes and occur over the course of several years—sometimes four or more, though they can last for as long as twenty years.

Hot flashes are extremely subjective. For some women, they happen around once a day, sometimes less. Some unlucky people have multiple hot flashes a day. How intense they are isn't universal, either. For some, they're a quick flush and a little heat; for others, they're much more intense. And that, of course, contributes to how disruptive they are for each individual.

Hot flashing at night, aka night sweats, is a real buzzkill. It's part of the reason so many people report sleep disruptions during menopause. If you've ever woken up with soaked pajamas and sheets, you've experienced night sweats. We're going to talk more in this chapter about sleep disruptions during menopause, and obviously hot flashing is a huge part of that.

I see you raising your hand! Your question is whether hot flashes can be a sign of cancer. The short answer is yes; *however*, if your night sweats are caused by cancer, the vast majority of the time, they're not the only symptom, according to the American Osteopathic Association. Among other things, they could be related to your thyroid. Doctors see an uptick in thyroid issues during this time, which can manifest themselves in some of the same symptoms. But you won't know for sure until you see an expert—and I absolutely do not mean Dr. Google. If you're experiencing more than usual fatigue, have lost weight without trying to, run fevers, or have unexplained pain, make an appointment with your doctor.

Tracking when your hot flashes happen will help inform what

you can do to lessen them. Think about whether consuming specific foods or beverages precedes a hot flash; spicy meals and alcohol can have an effect. Researchers from Liverpool John Moores University in the United Kingdom found that exercising can help reduce the frequency, as well as the severity and length, of hot flashes by helping the body with thermoregulation. More on that in part IV.

When Hot Flashes Meet the Real World

Sometimes a hot flashing woman just needs to get creative. We put that to the test by asking fellow menopausers how they've managed to control their hot flashing.

MC in New York City: "Hot flashes came on twice a day, on the hour-long subway ride in the crush of people to and from work. So I started carrying a huge Yeti thermos with the iciest ice cold water. When I felt one coming on, I'd put my hair on top of my head so it wasn't on my neck, take off any clothes I could manage to shed, and really go to town on that water. More than once I got off at the next stop and ran to the street level. In wintertime, this was a great fix. In the summer, I'd hail a taxi to take me the rest of the way home—and ask the driver to crank the AC."

LG in Highland Park, Illinois: "Yes, I get hot flashes, but I feel like I'm just constantly operating at a higher temperature than I was before. My fix? I carry around a handheld fan I bought off Amazon for about $8. I bring it with me everywhere, and I don't mind whipping it out whenever the heat comes—and boy, does it come. I bought about a dozen and have given them to my friends."

> **LL in Los Angeles:** "I purchased a cooling pad for my bed which pumps cold liquid through this membrane that sits on top of my mattress. It is igloo-like, and it is wonderful. Also expensive. Luckily, it covers only my half of my bed. My husband was not so keen on sleeping in an Arctic tundra."

Are Hot Flashes Dangerous?

For most women who have fairly typical hot flashes—as many as a couple a day for up to several years—they don't seem to be particularly risky. However, for women who are having significant hot flashes, meaning six or more a day, there seems to be a cardiovascular risk. A 2021 paper published in the *Journal of the American Heart Association* that was based on data collected in the Study of Women's Health Across the Nation (SWAN), one of the best long-term analyses of diverse women across the United States, found that among 3,083 women, most of whom were in their midforties and whom researchers had followed for up to twenty-two years, those with persistent vasomotor symptoms (hot flashing, flushed skin, sweating) had about a twofold greater chance of developing a cardiac event later in life, and as the severity and persistence of the hot flashes increased, so did the risk of cardiac events. As I'll get into later in the book, heart disease is the number one killer of women, yet doctors don't fully understand why that is. If we can come to understand why there's a link between a common menopause symptom and heart disease, in the future it may help us prevent loss of life. For now, if you are experiencing vasomotor symptoms that seem out of the ordinary, and *especially* if you have a family history of heart disease, link up with a cardiologist who can run tests and follow your trajectory as you make the menopause transition.

What Can I Do About Them?

Since the vast majority of people experiencing menopause end up tangoing with hot flashes, it's probably unsurprising that I spend a lot of my time talking about them. Over the course of thousands of conversations, I've learned a few things. They remain true when it comes to treating less top-of-mind and not so common symptoms, too. Here's my thinking. ·

◆ There are some really great medical options and some lackluster ones. Controversy over a poorly done study linking estrogen therapy to breast cancer has colored society's thinking about hormone replacement. There's a lot of nuance. There are treatments that will work for some people but not for others.

◆ There are some really great herbal and nonmedicinal options, and, like the medical ones, some are lackluster. Because of the way drugs are researched—based on which ones will have big paydays for the pharmaceutical companies that manufacture them—there are precious few studies that look at herbal medicine or other nondrug interventions, such as CBD, meditation, and acupuncture, for menopause symptoms. Overall, some treatments will work for some people but not for others.

I fully respect if you want to only go for prescriptions because you find natural food stores too woo-woo for your taste or they are inaccessible where you live. I fully respect if you want to try to exhaust over-the-counter or less conventional options first before your doctor whips out her prescription pad. Where I have fallen on this as a doctor is that there are some women whose symptoms are so severe and their quality of life is so diminished that it's dominating daily life and weighing down their mental health. For them, I would start a conversation about more conventional modes of treatment, which may include hormone therapy. There are other women who find their symptoms manageable but annoying and who want to improve how they're feeling both physically and emotionally but don't want to start with the heavy guns. And of course all of this changes if you have a history of hormone-receptive cancer, as I have, as opposed to someone without that or a family history.

I want to help my patients feel their best and do what's right for them during this transition, enabling them to thrive. I know I sound a bit like a motivational poster. But we've got to look out for one another! Let's thrive, damn it!

In order for us to understand our options, we have to do a quick history lesson about how we got to this place in gynecological medicine. I swear on a stack of *The Feminine Mystique* that it's not boring. It actually is emblematic of larger societal woes—and therefore forms the outline of what so many of us are fighting against.

Mainstream medicine has a woman problem, and the painful truth is that science fails us.

Since the time of the ancient Greeks, doctors have known that women respond differently to medicine than men. However, women have historically been, and often continue to be, excluded from clinical trials. Why is that? Menstruation. Researchers thought that it would be too hard to control for females' fluctuating hormone levels depending on where the participants were in their cycles.

I have to pause here for a minute and give some voice to a serious issue in medicine and the scientific community that studies people. In this diatribe, I'm going to talk about the binary terms "female" and "male." I do so because it is the distinction that is nearly universal in published research, except for studies that are specific to the trans community. This is, obviously, another shortcoming that the scientific community has yet to fully face. However, using the binary model helps explain why females have generally been underserved by Western medicine, which manifests itself in both physical and mental health.

Things get even worse if you're a female of color. I'm hopeful that identifying the patriarchal and White supremacist foundation persisting in medicine will open the door to representation not just for females but for all those who weren't born a White, cisgendered male.

This is painful for me because, as a dutiful member of Gen X, I was raised to believe that the best way to create change was from within the system. My duty as a privileged person was to work hard, move into spheres of influence and power via my access to the privileged, and then, *bam!*, lay it on them! By participating in what I naively perceived to be at least a partially merit-based system, my contributions would be recognized, valued, and accepted. I could work for change within the system. I don't even know if I believe that anymore, and it's rough. It's why I do this work speaking directly to the public and not isolating in an ivory tower. It's not enough to be a feminist salmon swimming upstream. And this salmon is *exhausted* by more than two decades of being seen as aggressive, bitchy, demanding, bossy, and intimidating instead of competent, responsible, admirable, and damn excellent at her job. Just this week, one of my favorite residents shared that she "loves me but the residents who don't work closely with me are afraid of me." It felt like a gut punch. The evidence on bias against women surgeons in the medical literature is mind boggling. The evidence on outcomes in any marginalized community—for instance, Black maternal mortality—is now well known and appalling.

I am far from throwing in the towel on changing the system from within, but it explains why I've never felt called to conventional academia. Instead, I have devoted myself to educating the public via media appearances, public speaking, and activities such as the Menopause Bootcamp. It is why I spend so much time building bridges between the integrative and conventional medical communities via teaching everyone from yoga therapy master's students at Loyola Marymount University to ob-gyn residents. It is why I keep listening so I can learn and share and do better. It is why this book includes many voices and lived experiences, not just those that reflect my own. I know I will get some of it wrong, and I ask that you understand that I, too, am human and am trying to serve you as best I can.

If you've ever been pregnant, you may have run into a medical question for which there's no clear answer. Whether to take a certain drug or undergo a procedure can feel like a crapshoot because there are little if any data to give you direction. Pregnant women are almost always excluded from studies that aren't pregnancy related. There are a couple reasons for that, including potential harm to the fetus or the pregnant person and the difficulty in parsing out whether an adverse effect—such as a miscarriage—is related to the drug being tested or if it's attributable to something else in the pregnancy (including natural causes). This issue was front and center when pregnant and lactating women were excluded from late-stage covid-19 vaccine trials. Of course, the drug companies don't want to put pregnant women and their fetuses at risk, and I'm certainly not suggesting that they should. In most drug trials, the criteria to be included in the early stages of early trials are a high bar, and pregnancy is almost always a reason for exclusion. On the other hand, by the time the last phases of drug research roll around, the drug's safety has already been established; animal studies, and then human studies, have sussed out the lion's share of side effects. By the last stage, researchers are establishing particularities such as dosage and frequency. If they wanted to, they could use their preexisting knowledge of similar drugs to determine whether it would be prudent to add pregnant or lactating people into a particular study. What happens when experts don't do that is what we saw during the covid pandemic. In the absence of research, ob-gyns like me were left to make educated decisions. A lot of us ended up participating in ad hoc registries and databases spearheaded by doctors at academic institutions. Once there was enough information to facilitate responsible recommendations, information was disseminated in a grassroots manner to practicing colleagues via the governing bodies of women's health medicine and to our patients via word of mouth and social media.

I think it's fair to say that the covid-19 vaccines are an exceptional case—fortunately, it's not every day that drug companies have to race to produce a silver bullet designed to be administered the world over. But the trials were closely watched by the public, which is far from the norm. Seldom do we celebrate those who are willing to be among the first to try an experimental treatment. The problem is, women are not asked often enough. "The under-representation of women in clinical trials stems from the long-held assumption that the male perspective represents the norm," wrote Rachel Brazil in a feature titled "Why We Need to Talk About Sex and Clinical Trials" in the *Pharmaceutical Journal*. "Medical education textbooks typically default to the male in case studies and anatomical drawings, while women are represented only in matters specific to reproductive biology." She went on to say, "It has become increasingly apparent that the male response to medicines does not represent both sexes. Rather than protecting women, evidence shows their exclusion from trials has led to an unrepresentative assessment of drug efficacy and side effects, potentially leaving them at risk of serious harm."

Consider this 2020 review from UC Berkeley and the University of Chicago: a review of thousands of research studies "found clear evidence of a drug dose gender gap for 86 different medications approved by the Federal Drug Administration (FDA), including antidepressants, cardiovascular and anti-seizure drugs and analgesics [painkillers], among others," according to a summary from the universities. The researchers found that after both genders were given the same dosage of one of those medications, blood tests revealed that women had higher concentrations of it in their systems, and it took longer for it to be eliminated. And they were way more likely to have stronger side effects, such as upset stomachs, headaches, depression, and heart issues. The research, led by Irving Zucker, a professor emeritus of psychology and integrative biology at UC Berkeley, and Brian Prender-gast, a psychologist at the University of Chicago, highlighted the drug zolpidem, aka Ambien. When women were given the same dosage that men were given (because the drug trials had used men to figure out how much should go into a pill), it stuck around in women's systems longer and they woke up groggier—so much so that it led to an in-crease in traffic accidents. The FDA was forced to reduce the dosage of zolpidem for women by half. Which is good, certainly. But it took a bunch of fatigued zombie women and a spate of traffic accidents to get there. And that's just one drug; one very lucrative, oft-prescribed drug. There are hundreds of drugs on the market, including chemotherapy drugs, that are not calibrated for women because there were no women subjects in the original drug trials, and the differences in side effects don't rise to such urgency that the FDA is going to review them for gender disparities.

Though the world of drug development isn't my area of expertise, I wanted to give you a sense of what exactly we're up against when it comes to understanding women's health. But it does set the stage for something that *is* in my wheelhouse, which is the available drugs for premenopausal and menopausal people. There simply are not nearly enough drugs being developed and studied for people who are going through the menopausal transition. And the research that is available isn't totally reliable.

Why Do We Have Such a Negative Reaction to Hormone Therapy?

Then there are times when research studies are focused on women and things go horribly wrong. Let me tell you a story that starts with three controversial words: menopausal hormone therapy.

When I bring up the topic of hormone therapy to patients, some of them get squeamish. I can tell that they're having a visceral reaction to the idea. Over the years, I've gathered that some of this is due to misinformation from other physicians who themselves are undereducated or otherwise uncomfortable with the treatment. Or these patients may have adopted the beliefs of an older generation that hormone replacement was dangerous and that it was an express train to things such as breast cancer and heart disease.

The pivot point for hormone replacement therapy, when a silver bullet turned into hemlock, came in July 2002. Up to that point, it seemed as though all women "of a certain age" were on menopausal hormone therapy. It was de rigueur for maintaining what was considered to be youthfulness. But that summer was when the Women's Health Initiative, a multicenter task force, published the results of its research in the *Journal of the American Medical Association*. The study looked at whether estrogen derived from horses (really) plus progestin caused health risks among the 8,506 people who had taken it versus the 8,102 women who had taken a placebo. The results were *stark*. "The primary outcome was coronary heart disease . . . with invasive breast cancer as the primary adverse outcome," the study authors wrote. "A global index summarizing the balance of risks and benefits included the 2 primary outcomes plus stroke, pulmonary embolism (PE), endometrial cancer, colorectal cancer, hip fracture, and death due to other causes." That was the medical equivalent of yelling "Fire!" in a crowded theater. It sent everybody running for the exits.

The study came out a year and a half after I graduated residency. I remember sitting in ob-gyn grand rounds, a weekly departmental conference, thinking about hormone replacement therapy, as we called it then, and how it was having so many positive effects on women, particularly their cardiovascular health. The Women's Health Initiative was a record scratch. HRT party over. Internists were pulling patients off prescriptions. The patients were flipping out about getting cancer or having a heart attack, and who could blame them?

Pretty quickly, we realized that the study was flawed. The average age of the test subjects was sixty-five, so they were ten years past the menopausal transition, when they had started taking hormones. A lot of them had a preexisting heart condition, which in and of itself made them bad candidates for this kind of therapy. And the most damning part was that the study had used the hormones Premarin and Provera, which are not actually one-to-one replacement hormones for what your body makes. (For what it's worth, we're not talking about some weird Franken-pharma concoction that was used injudiciously—at the time, these were two of the most widely prescribed drugs.) The hormones replaced hormones lost due to menopause with *hormones your body doesn't naturally make*. The conclusion we clinicians draw from this study now isn't that hormones are actually 100 percent safe; it's that the data can't be applied as broadly as we had expected or hoped.

In the two decades since, science has been walking back the data. Because, yes, for some people, menopausal hormone therapy is a bad idea owing to their health record or family history. But something interesting happened, too: the Women's Health Initiative study created a vacuum of options for women. And what ended up filling that vacuum is bioidentical hormones and alternative therapies.

We did get some good information from the study, including data showing that women who had had a hysterectomy had a lower risk of developing breast cancer, meaning that the line between hormones (or lack thereof) and health is not always predictable. And I want to pull out one other takeaway that's relevant to you reading this today, which is that patients need to be assessed individually. Even if the study had turned out differently, the lesson should still have been that there's no such thing as a blanket prescription. All of my patients are unique, and the complexity of who they are is determined by genetics, their health history, and their present state of health—including their diets, activity levels, and mental health.

I don't know what the motivation was behind giving everyone

hormone replacement therapy at the time. The promise of youth forever? Suppression of aging? Today, we are much more thoughtful
about how we prescribe menopausal hormone therapy. There are people it'll help and people it'll hurt, and that can be assessed in a medically responsible way by considering the nuances of a patient's medical
makeup.

Two More Hot Topics in Menopausal Hormone Therapy

Why I Do Not Recommend Pellets for Anyone

For the uninitiated, pellets are small testosterone or estrogen pellets
the size of a grain of rice that are injected into a person's buttock. The
scuttlebutt among some of my patients is that they are a kind of
fountain of youth, making them feel energized and decreasing some
of their symptoms of menopause (hot flashes, mood swings, dry
vagina, energy level, libido, and others). But pellets don't work for
everyone. Among some people, they cause major side effects or complications, including abnormal bleeding, acne, clitoral enlargement,
hair changes, mood issues, heart problems; basically, they can create
supraphysiological levels of estrogen and testosterone, and some of the
negative side effects can be permanent. The pellets aren't removable, so
you have to wait three to six months for the effects of the hormones
to diminish. Also, there is that pesky hole in your butt where the pellet
was inserted. I don't recommend them for anyone.

What Are Bioidentical Hormones, and Why Do
People Get Mad About Them?

Our quest to go all natural has seeped into hormone treatment.
Proponents of bioidentical hormones say that they're healthier than
and superior to "lab-made" hormones. This is a bit of magical thinking. As I say to my patients, unless you are willing to kill the person

next to you, harvest her ovaries, and use them as your menopausal hormone therapy, there's nothing natural about your MHT.

Let's take these two questions separately.

What are bioidentical hormones? You'd think this would be an easy question to answer, but according to a 2011 paper in the journal *Mayo Clinic Proceedings*, "The term *bioidentical hormone* does not have a standardized definition and thus often confuses patients and practitioners." It went on to say:

> Women who request bioidentical HT [hormone therapy] (BHT) from their physicians may have differing expectations. Depending on the circumstances, it can mean natural (not artificial), compounded, plant derived, or chemically identical to the human hormone structure. The Endocrine Society has defined bioidentical hormones as "compounds that have exactly the same chemical and molecular structure as hormones that are produced in the human body." This broad definition does not address the manufacturing, source, or delivery methods of the products and thus can include non–FDA-approved custom-compounded products as well as FDA-approved formulations.

It's frustrating to define something by defining what it's not. But I hope that while reading this, you are picking up on the confusion that swirls around bioidentical hormone therapy. Bioidentical, as the word suggests, means that the hormones are chemically identical to the hormones your body produces on its own. What you have to understand is that the chemicals in bioidentical hormone meds are often identical to those in traditional hormone therapy.

Earlier we talked about the importance of language, which is something that comes up in medicine a lot. It's important to acknowledge that both the American College of Obstetricians and Gynecologists and the Endocrine Society have stated that bioidentical hormone replacement therapy is not a standard term and is, instead, a marketing device, but I disagree. It is a description of how the medications are made up, and it encompasses a fair amount of FDA-approved options for menopausal hormone therapy (MHT). *All* of them are manufactured in a factory and probably get their base products from some of the same vendors. The difference is that pharmaceutical companies have to adhere to strict FDA processing regulations regarding dosages and the ratios of hormones in their products and makers of bioidentical HRTs have more leeway.

Yes, it's true that some non-FDA-approved—and even some FDA-approved—compounded MHTs are plant derived. But though it seems to make a lot more sense to "replace" a hormone with something as close as possible to what is now diminished, their being "natural" does not necessarily make them superior.

Why do people get mad about them? In the wake of the Women's Health Initiative report, people continued to enter menopause and continued to feel all the same signs and symptoms they had previously. Only now they had weighty questions about how best to manage them and move into the next phase healthily. Additionally, enormous and valid issues of trust were unearthed by the massive failure on the part of the medical establishment to protect women and preserve our health. Only nine years previously, the FDA had acknowledged the shortcomings of most twentieth-century medical research and committed to including women in research and specifically addressing drugs' impacts on women. The vacuum left by the Women's Health Initiative debacle was filled with alternatives.

I believe that this is one of the defining moments in modern women's health. It resulted in the rise of so-called bioidenticals, created by compounding pharmacies that were making custom-tailored MHT—and Suzanne Somers as the spokesperson for "how to properly menopause." Let me just pause (ahem) for a moment here to acknowledge and thank Ms. Somers for her audacity in embracing her personal brand of aging. Let's face it, *no one* was talking about aging out loud in polite company or admitting they were experiencing it when she published her number one bestseller *Ageless: The Naked Truth About Bioidentical Hormones* in 2006. Her use of bioidentical hormone replacement therapy (BHRT) became de rigueur for many who sought out the newest and latest, and they were off to the races.

There were some doctors who saw an opportunity to serve and others who identified an opportunity to charge for a needed service that insurance didn't deem worthy of much reimbursement; a forty-minute, insurance-paid consult doesn't pay enough to keep an office open long, but testing hormones and selling from your own on-site pharmacy does! It was around that time that I, too, took it upon myself to get educated. The Women's Health Initiative report had kicked me in the ass, too! It had shaken my core beliefs in the monolith of science, truth, and medicine. I will say that my early forays into some of the less conventional educational conferences were much more science based than I'd anticipated, but they were also pretty out there.

Here is what I can tell you—and what was echoed in a 2017 study published in the journal *BMC Women's Health* of reasons why women choose BHRT. Menopausal people are wary of conventional medicine due to mistrust, bad experiences when they were not heard, and their concerns not being addressed or taken seriously, as well as significant concerns about safety that the media reported over and over. They are pulled toward alternatives such as compounded BHRTs because the products are made out to be more natural or safer and provide many more ways to treat than do the standard FDA-approved MHT offerings, which currently include patches, pills, gels, sprays, vaginal tablets, creams, rings, and suppositories—though far fewer options were available in the early 2000s.

Compounders can provide a wider variety of dosages, combinations of multiple hormones, and methods of dispensing the hormones such as lozenges, under-the-tongue tinctures, creams, lotions, and pills. The issues of regulatory oversight, lack of standardization, safety, and efficacy are, however, valid. I am fortunate to work in a large city where I know my pharmacists personally and have access to their high-integrity practices and protocols. I do not sell anything in my practice, so my motivation is merely to help my patients get the best that is available. My go-to is always FDA-approved products first, and then, if they are not working or acceptable, we can move—safely, I believe—to compounded BHRT. But I don't trust the all-or-nothing, scorched-earth approach of those who absolutely reject any and all alternatives. It is an attitude of paternalism: "I know what's best for you." That smacks of a lack of willingness to read, listen, grow, and evolve. What's needed is lifelong learning.

* * *

So that takes us back to where we started: hot flashes. After all, the first FDA-approved estrogen product, Premarin, was approved to treat that very symptom. The road to FDA-approved drugs for menopausal symptoms has been fraught, when there's been a road at all. I wish I could say that there are exciting new drugs on the horizon, but I'd be lying. There aren't many more options now than there were five or ten years ago, and I don't expect that that will change in the near future. The drugs that are available have checkered histories and often insufficient data to support them. I'm not suggesting that doctors are playing a guessing game, but I will say that I wish drug companies were as concerned about the physical encumbrances of menopausal women as they are about erectile dysfunction. I'm not even being glib. I'm glad that ED drugs are tested and available. I just want women to be afforded the same respect. If you're thinking to yourself, "Suzanne, I just thought of something funny: the physical and sexual well-being of men over fifty is paramount, while women over fifty are desexualized and overlooked," you and I are on the same wavelength. And we're going to get there! But there's going to be a Menopause Bootcamp mutiny if I don't finally tell you what in God's name to do about your hellish hot flashes.

It's imperative that I tell you one last thing before I get to those treatment options, because it's really at the heart of my thinking on menopause. When the full weight of what I described—the facts that women are excluded by design from medical research that affects both genders and female-specific medical needs are not being adequately met by the drug companies—sank in, I felt awful for my patients, my friends, and even myself. It's discriminatory, plain and simple. And although I assume that some slow changes are taking place in the pharmaceutical industry, these are problems we've been dealing with for decades, so I'm not holding my breath that there'll be a sea change in my professional lifetime. When I look for the sorts of top-shelf studies that doctors depend on—ones that use sufficiently large participant pools and are peer reviewed—I often come up short. So I'm left trying methods on my patients that are not backed by the same kind of rigorous academic research afforded to pharmaceutical-grade drugs but do have historical usage in complementary medicine along with patient testimonials.

That was one of the big reasons I turned to Ayurveda and other alternative therapies. I'll be honest, they are not all FDA approved. They may also have smaller studies backing them up, often done outside of the United States, Western Europe, and the comfort zone of some. Or anecdotal evidence and logical leaps may play into our decision to try out a treatment. Again, for the majority of generally healthy patients, there's trial and error. If something doesn't move the needle, we can move on. This holds true for both Western and Eastern treatments.

The Main Event: How to Deal with Those F@#$ing Hot Flashes

We're going to break this down into three parts: prescription drugs, over-the-counter drugs and herbs, and lifestyle changes. Here's how to use this list.

The first thing I set out to do with any patient is simple: I need to hear your story in your own words. This helps us identify your priorities and set goals. What's bothering you the most, and what do you hope to change, feel, or improve? This enables us to explore and activate solutions based on your specific history (you were an emotional wreck when you were on birth control pills or had endometriosis), risk factors (you had cancer or have high blood pressure or all the women in your family wind up with dementia and Alzheimer's), and particular needs (you love to run marathons and miss having sex with your partner).

The other pearl here is what I call "applying tincture of time"—otherwise known as good old-fashioned patience. There is *no* way anyone can get answers to everything all at once. Over many years in medical practice, I have learned that if we attempt to do too much at one time, you will feel overwhelmed and may not do anything we planned on. Moreover, initiating too many changes at once will obscure their individual results, and we won't know what is actually effective. I also do triage. In other words, what *must* be dealt with first in order to impact anything else? Usually it's sleep. If we don't repair your sleep, your mood, thinking, sex—in fact, your entire life—is not going to work. Often hot flashes are the source of sleep deprivation, so I do start there. But honestly, if I had to pick one priority that is common to everyone, it would be the restoration of a sense of well-being. The loss of our sense of self, agency in our lives, and the ability to function is huge, and if we can work toward solving those problems, you will know that what I say is true: "It really will be not just okay but quite possibly great!"

Prescription Drugs for Hot Flashes

Mood Stabilizers/Antidepressants

A review of research published in *Journal of General Internal Medicine* encompassing eleven randomized controlled trials found that among women going through the menopause transition and after, selective serotonin reuptake inhibitors (SSRIs) can reduce the frequency and severity of hot flashes. They may not be good for women with high blood pressure and some shouldn't be taken by women who have had breast cancer and take tamoxifen.

Menopause Hormone Therapy

This is a low-dose hormone therapy that replaces some of the estrogen that's lost during the menopausal transition. The loss of hormones is the driving force of hot flashes, so compensating for some of that hormone loss has a positive effect on hot flashes. Whether it's right for you will depend on your family history, genetic predispositions, and health status, as well as what you're hoping to use it for. Additionally, progestin or my preference, progesterone, is used in those with a uterus to protect from overstimulating it with estrogen.

Gabapentin

Typically prescribed to control seizures due to epilepsy, as well as reduce pain owing to nerve damage, the drug gabapentin is also prescribed for some to help with hot flashes. For some, side effects such as drowsiness, fatigue, dizziness, and water retention in the limbs occur, so they discontinue it. But for others, it at least somewhat improves their flashing without much, if any, downside. While we're here, I'll mention that I don't like to prescribe clonidine, which is a sedative and also used to treat hypertension. It's an old drug with potential side effects, and I think there are better options.

Over-the-Counter Supplements and Herbs for Hot Flashes

Everything in this list is fairly easy to buy in the United States, either in natural food stores or online. I am particular about safety and recommend only particular brands for that reason. My favorites include Enzymedica, Mountain Rose Herbs, Metagenics, Banyan Botanicals, Vital Nutrients, Remifemin, Kindra, and Cannapy Health. One of the big criticisms of herbal medicine is that it's not regulated by the Food and Drug Administration and therefore doesn't have to meet the same standards as pharmaceuticals that are prescribed or sold over the counter, such as aspirin and Benadryl. The Dietary Supplement Health and Education Act of 1984 does regulate these products but with less rigor than the FDA does pharmaceuticals. That is why I am so particular about the brands I recommend and use myself, because they have been vetted for safety and efficacy.

I'll be honest with you: there are not as many research studies to attest to herbal medicines' efficacy compared with pharmaceuticals. You can probably figure out the biggest reason: money. The medical-industrial complex puts billions of research dollars into testing prescription drugs and treatments, for which they can earn a lot of sales revenue, and there's not nearly as much potential profit in herbal medicines. But the limitations of medical evidence for botanicals does not need to be a reason to avoid trying them. There is enough evidence about their safety. And for the most part, their side effects are less extreme than they are for many pharmaceutical drugs. Unlike pharma solutions, they will take longer to work—typically thirty to ninety days—and require consistent use as directed. I'm going to try to educate you about the options available and which may work for you, but you have to be patient; it may take a while to feel the effects. If you have questions, talk to your doctor and possibly an herbalist, who can guide you through remedies for the symptoms you have.

As a board-certified ob-gyn and integrative women's health doctor and a breast cancer survivor, these are my tried-and-true natural product–based solutions. Remember that when using supplements, you should make sure that they don't interact with any medications you are already taking.

Black Cohosh

This is a plant that's native to North America; the supplement extract is made from the roots and underground stems. There have been a number of studies over the years that have tried to validate the effectiveness of black cohosh, and they've been a mixed bag. But a lot of my patients have found relief using it for up to six months. Black cohosh seems to be safe for people taking other medications, though it may change the efficacy of statins, according to researchers at the University of North Carolina. The dosage is 20 milligrams twice a day.

Red Clover

This herb, which is part of the legume family and boasts red flowers, is found in Asia, Europe, and North America. Red clover's effectiveness for menopause symptoms is probably due to its isoflavones, which act as a phytoestrogen (much like soy). For the same reason, red clover may be useful for staving off osteoporosis. But those with a history of breast cancer should avoid it. It's available in tea, capsule, extract, and tincture forms, as well as topical form for some skin issues. Follow the packaging directions for dosage.

Soy Isoflavones

Like red clover, the soybean is a legume, and its isoflavones are effective among some people who are dealing with night sweats and hot flashes. A 2019 paper in the journal *Nutrients* suggested that soy isoflavones may reduce the risk of developing certain cancers and other diseases. Forty to 80 milligrams per day of commercially prepared isoflavones are usually recommended. The data are mostly inconclusive, but it's worth a try. Because soy-based medicines are thought to act like estrogens, there is some controversy in its use among breast cancer survivors. Some data, especially those from studies that investigated soy-heavy diets, including in Japan, indicate a reduction in breast cancer risk. And in vitro (lab-based) science explorations of how these plant chemicals, used for millennia by many cultures, work in the body have indicated potent anticancer benefits. But, "While there is no clear evidence of harm, better evidence confirming safety is required before use of high dose (≥100 mg) isoflavones can be recommended in breast cancer patients," according to researchers at the Canadian College of Naturopathic Medicine and others.

Evening Primrose Oil

Evening primrose oil comes from the Americas and is special for its content of gamma-linolenic acid (GNA), an essential fatty acid. Evening primrose oil has been used to treat premenstrual breast pain, as have other omega-3 fatty acids. Presumably these oils work by exerting an anti-inflammatory effect. In some small randomized trials, 1,000 milligrams twice a day of evening primrose oil has been shown to reduce the frequency and severity of night sweats.

Russian or Siberian Rhubarb

This plant has been used for millennia by Chinese and European herbalists. Modern science has demonstrated that it acts like a selective estrogen receptor modulator (SERM), according to a paper published in the journal *Chinese Medicine*; it selectively binds to some estrogen B receptors and has been shown in several small trials to calm hot flashes but not to increase endometrial tissue proliferation, which could lead to cancer. It seems for this reason to be safe for breast cancer survivors, but it might compete with tamoxifen and other estrogen-dependent cancer treatments, so it should be used with caution and under the supervision of a knowledgeable physician.

Pycnogenol/French Marine Pine Bark Extract

This fascinating botanical, derived from, yes, pine bark, is grown in the Mediterranean area and, according to the menopause journalist Ann Marie McQueen, is processed in a standardized and safe manner in Europe. You have probably never heard of it, and neither had I until recently. It is the key ingredient in one of my favorite supplements made by Kindra. I love it so much that not only do I take it daily, but I joined Kindra's Scientific Advisory Board! This plant-based medicine has a multitude of anti-inflammatory effects, which explains its benefits for cardiometabolic and brain health as well as arthritis, in addition to hot flashes—though how it works on that is unknown. Two hundred milligrams per day to 300 milligrams twice a day are common safe doses.

Milk Thistle

This is a very popular herbal preparation most often thought of in connection with "liver cleansing" (a term I typically avoid as it is not used in conventional medicine and triggers all sorts of mayhem and judgments!). It must be used with care, as it can activate a liver enzyme (cytochrome P450) that is involved in processing medications and cause drug interactions. But it has shown promise in the treatment of osteoporosis and reduction of hot flashes in some small recent trials over a three-month period of time. The dose is 400 milligrams per day for twelve weeks.

Vitamin E

This occurs naturally in many foods, including olive oil, almonds, peanuts, and leafy greens, but it's also a good supplement to add to your diet. In addition to calming hot flashes, vitamin E is important for your brain, blood, vision, and skin. Aim to get 15 milligrams of vitamin E per day. A small trial using high doses of 200 to 500 milligrams per day over a two- to four-month period resulted in minimal impact, and as these doses can also theoretically increase bleeding, it seems as though the risk of taking a higher dose does not outweigh the benefits.

The Power of CBD

I want to talk about this separately because I'm a big believer in it for many symptoms of menopausal and even nonmenopausal symptoms. CBD, or cannabidiol, is the nonpsychoactive part of the cannabis plant; its counterpart that gets you high is THC. It comes in many different forms, including tinctures, gummies, vapes, and capsules, all of which are taken orally, as well as topical creams, gels, lotions, and oils—even lube. It seems to have positive effects on hot flashes, sleep, mood, and more. The reason it could possibly be effective for hot flashes boils down to its ability in some people to modulate stress and anxiety. We know that those are triggers of hot flashes, and if CBD can keep you in a calmer state, it stands to reason that your hot flashes may also be kept at bay. It could also be that CBD has a more direct effect on hot flashes, by modulating the thermoregulation systems that are thrown off during the menopausal transition—but not enough research has been done up to now to know one way or another. Now, CBD doesn't affect everyone the same way, so, as with all of my recommendations, what works for your friend may not work for you. But generally speaking, it's worth a shot.

Lifestyle Changes

Make Exercise Part of Your Routine

There's good science to suggest that hot-flashing women who follow a regular exercise routine see a reduction in episodes and severity.

In a 2016 study published in the journal *Menopause*, researchers surveyed twenty-one postmenopausal women about their hot flashes and put them through fitness testing, then guided them through either a sixteen-week exercise program or a control condition. Those who moved their bodies during those four months had better cardiorespiratory fitness and improved their hot flashes more than the control group. It's probably because exercise helps thermoregulation—the body's internal thermostat, which is thrown off during menopause—coupled with better blood flow and sweating efficiency. The benefits of exercise are going to pop up at many points from here on out, because there are so many benefits for both physical and mental health. If you're just getting back into exercise after being away from it for a while, it's best to start slowly. If your first foray is to a forty-five-minute crazy bootcamp, you may actually find that it triggers hot flashes. The thermoregulatory benefits are something that you will develop over time, so limit the intensity and build up your stamina with longer bouts of exercise. Think walking or jogging, hiking, biking, rowing or kayaking, yoga, elliptical, Pilates, swimming—basically, anything you enjoy and have access to. Once you can comfortably go thirty minutes and feel strong and comfortable, and the exercise is not triggering hot flashes, try to increase the intensity. If you're hot flashing or you feel as though it takes a really long time for your core body temperature to go back down and that's bothersome, ratchet down either the time or the effort. And don't forget to go at your own speed! Remember, all of this should be highly personalized to you. And you're playing the long game! Rather than racing to improve your fitness in the next two weeks, think about where you want to be six months or a year from now.

Drink Ice-Cold Water

Doing this is like creating a direct line to reducing your core body temperature. Sip a big glass of ice water over a minute or two when a hot flash begins. Some patients find it helpful to keep an insulated bottle of ice water at their bedside to nip a night sweat in the bud.

Reduce Your Alcohol Intake—Probably

For some people, hooch is an express train to hot flashes. There's not a lot of research behind this, but it may be due to the fact that alcohol causes an inflammatory response in the body, which raises the internal body temperature. Back when you were premenopausal, your body's thermoregulation worked well enough to cope. Postmenopause, the temperature change that alcohol causes throws everything out of whack. Plus, alcohol is a sleep disruptor; its depressant qualities may knock you out, but they mess up your normal sleep cycle, and once the depressant wears off in the middle of the night, you can find yourself wide awake and unable to get back to sleep. Plus, alcohol usage over time causes chronic inflammation, leading to metabolic disorders and other diseases such as cancer. Talking solely about hot flashes, though, if you notice that the nights you drink have you sweating through your PJs, try laying off the booze for two weeks and see what effect it has on your thermoregulation.

In my research for this book, I also found that for some people, alcohol has the opposite effect, and I think it's only fair to bring it up. Research from the University of Maryland, Mercy Medical Center in Baltimore, Johns Hopkins University School of Medicine, and the University of Illinois found that in perimenopause, at least, alcohol may have a mediating effect, possibly because of the bump it causes in blood glucose. So where do I come down on the alcohol question? Well, alcohol disrupts sleep, which has downstream health effects. And it causes inflammation—and for some people chronic inflammation, which is dangerous. At the same time, giving up alcohol entirely isn't something that everyone wants to do. For them, I'd say certainly don't drink for the prevention of hot flashes alone. There are other methods that don't carry risks. And if you keep the drinking in check, save for an occasional glass of wine with friends or beer at a ball game, adding up to no more than one to three drinks per week *depending on your individual health risks*, it's probably okay. But if you have a personal or family history of breast cancer, I suggest that you cut your drinking back to as close to zero as possible.

Stop Smoking

Smoking is linked to hot flashes and a thousand other terrible things. I know you know this, and I'm not here to lecture you and make you feel bad. But please, try like hell to stop smoking. In the last several years, the FDA has approved new smoking cessation drugs that have been game changers, even for lifelong smokers who have tried unsuccessfully to put down the cigs in the past. The American Lung Association (www.lung.org) has great resources, including support groups. You've got this.

Give Acupuncture a Go

In the past several years, acupuncture has enjoyed more mainstream acceptance in the West, but it's been a cornerstone of traditional Chinese medicine for centuries. Part of why it's gaining traction here in the United States is that studies are confirming its efficacy for treating a range of conditions, including hot flashes. Research published in the journal *Menopause* in 2016 described a yearlong study involving 209 perimenopausal and postmenopausal women, ages forty-five to sixty. All of them reported having four or more vasomotor symptoms a day, including hot flashes, daytime or night sweats, and flushing, and were assigned to have twenty acupuncture treatments over the course of six months. Half of the participants got them for the first six months of the study, half of them the second six months. The women who were needled first saw their vasomotor symptoms drop by almost 37 percent, whereas the women who were waiting for their turn had an increase of 6 percent. The positive effects lasted at least six months after the acupuncture treatments ended. Best of all, the women reported improvements in their overall quality of life.

I'm guessing that there were study participants for whom the techniques worked amazingly, and others who experienced little change. But that's fine! It's what we would expect. We're able to say "no harm, no foul" because if you're going to a reputable practitioner, there are zero side effects. Acupuncture is done by locating spots on the body where there may be energy blockages; that's how acupuncturists talk about it. And when you go, they may insert needles to help with hot flashes, as well as stress, gastrointestinal issues, or low energy.

I've done acupuncture on and off over the years myself. I think one of the reasons I go back to it is its meditative quality. Picture this: You're lying on a table either faceup or facedown. The needles take a few nearly painless minutes to place. Now your job is to sit quietly and very, very still while listening to calming spa music for thirty minutes to an hour. That in and of itself is healing. No work calls. No texts from your kids asking you what you're making for dinner. No distraction. Just meditation. We need to learn to schedule time for ourselves that is nonnegotiable. After all, we are such active listeners to the needs of others and are socially trained to be tireless caretakers of everyone but ourselves. We deserve care, too.

Dear reader, would you excuse me for a sec while I book an acupuncture appointment?

I Love the Placebo Effect (and You Should, Too)

There's a misconception that doctors aren't fans of the placebo effect. To refresh your memory, a placebo is a research tool. It's used as a control to test the efficacy of the drug or procedure that the scientists are actually trying to test. In popular culture (and often in research settings), it's a sugar pill. For instance, if you're testing the effectiveness of a new antidepressant, half of the people are given that new drug, and half are given a placebo. Sometimes, by the end of the study, the people taking the real drug do a lot better. Other times, neither group improves much (meaning that the drug wasn't effective). But a surprising number of times, researchers find that the new drug they are testing was effective, *and the group taking the placebo improved, too!* It's proof that the mind-body connection is strong. If you're a participant in that study, you have depressive symptoms that you want to reduce. Taking that pill is proactive and a form of self-care—regardless if it's medicine or not. And believe it or not, research suggests that the placebo effect can work *even when the person knows that what he or she is taking is a placebo.*

One doctor I admire greatly, Dr. Wayne Jonas, who's a board-certified family physician and expert in integrative health, says that the placebo effects that occur in many clinical research efforts are likely attributable, in part, to what he calls "meaning and context." If the goal is healing or restoration of well-being, does it matter what caused the improvement? As long as there is no evidence of harm, a placebo is acceptable and possibly even helpful. This is the guiding principle in my own practice and teaching.

The placebo effect also helps explain people who are into healing stones. If you know about crystal healing, you've heard that rose quartz can instill peace and emotional healing. If you want those things, you might ascribe a rose quartz rock with those powers. And if picking up the stone is the catalyst for that self-healing and peace—well, I say that's pretty awesome.

I assume you know that I'm not saying that you should eschew chemotherapy for crystals. I'm saying you can use both. You may recall the story I told you in the introduction to this book about DD, the patient I had during residency who adorned her hospital room with Tibetan flags and asked me to dab on essential oils for clarity before I took part in the team that performed her surgery. The surgery went great, and she healed extraordinarily quickly. Our minds are absolutely connected to our bodies and vice versa. Denying that is bad for both doctors and patients.

Explore Cognitive Behavioral Therapy (CBT)

It seems that when it comes to hot flashes and night sweats, there's an emotional component. Anxiety and stress are contributing forces, which is why researchers at the Robert Wood Johnson Medical School did a pilot study in the mid-2000s that found that CBT—a form of talk therapy that helps you identify unhelpful thought patterns and learn how to better respond to challenging or uncomfortable situations—can be effective in reducing hot flashes. This reveals two ways in which anxiety or stress can trigger a hot flash. In the first, something happens—you get into a fender bender, and the driver of the other car storms over and starts yelling—and that triggers vasomotor symptoms. Another pathway is anxiety over the hot flash itself. For a lot of women, they come on so often and so strongly that the mere thought of them is scary, and that triggers a hot flash— because of course it does. CBT can teach you methods of thinking that make it so that fear over hot flashing doesn't become a self-fulfilling prophecy.

Try Essential Oils

Using your index finger, dab a small amount of a cooling or calming essential oil—eucalyptus, lavender, peppermint, sandalwood, spearmint, or vetiver, among others—to clean, dry skin at the top of your forehead, behind your ears, or along the back of your neck. These body points are rich in blood supply, and the oils may help to cool you off.

Curb Your Intake of Spicy Food and Caffeine

I love both of these and am not recommending complete abstinence, but a lot of women experience an increase in hot flashes as a result of consuming spicy food and caffeine-containing beverages. Although caffeine is a vasoconstrictor, it can result in an increased heart rate, which can trigger a hot flash. If you love it, you may have to deal with some increased hot flashing. That's an example of the trade-offs we make when we want to do things that aren't always good for us but make us happy. If you want to stick to a happy medium, order the spicy curry and double cappuccino in January, when it's cold anyway, and eschew spice and caffeine when it's August and a hot flash is around every corner.

Pretend That It's Summer

Whatever you do to keep cool during the summer will work for a hot flash: wearing light clothing or layers that you can pull off, holding a cold pack to the back of your neck or your wrist, sleeping on performance bed sheets that keep you cooler, using a handheld fan—anything to make those moments more comfortable.

Sleep Disruption (Home Shopping Network's 3:00 A.M. Time Slot Just Got a New Viewer)

I remember the first night I woke up and my pajamas were soaked through. The sheets, too. It's not surprising that people's first thought is often that they wet the bed. The whole thing is superupsetting, and it's another really common complaint. According to the Sleep Foundation, about 12 percent of premenopausal women have sleep issues, and that number jumps to 40 percent among women in their forties and early fifties. Hot flashes and night sweats, insomnia—the inability to fall asleep—and midsleep disruption crop up a lot among my patients, as do new diagnoses of sleep apnea and restless legs syndrome or periodic limb movements disorder. And when you've been sleeping poorly for a couple days or weeks, you end up slogging through your daytime and fearing the nights of tossing and turning. The lack of sleep and the anxiety it causes can lead to depression.

One quick note: The other major reason you might be getting up throughout the night is to go to the bathroom. Frequent urination is a huge sleep disruption issue. It has to do with decreasing levels of a hormone called vasopressin, which regulates our ability to sleep through the night with a full bladder without wetting ourselves. That hormone diminishes with age, and there is no replacement therapy for it. Decreasing or eliminating your alcohol consumption at night, stopping your caffeine intake after noon, and improving your overall sleep hygiene are ways you can improve this menopausal phenomenon.

Because hot flashes are related to sleep disruptions, the fixes for the first also apply to the second. For treating sleep specifically, I usually recommend behavioral changes before meds, some of which I'll go through.

Exercise in the Morning Rather than at Night

If you're a frequent exerciser, you probably have a favorite time of day to pump iron or go the distance. That may have to do with your chronotype, which is a concept meaning your body's specific internal clock. However, one thing to watch out for is your core body temperature when you go to bed. We know that exercise makes you heat up, something that's especially true if you're doing intensive training or working out in the heat. Your body may need more time to get back to a cooler temperature than it did when you were premenopausal.

Address Your So-Called Sleep Hygiene

This has been a buzzy term in the past few years ever since Arianna Huffington told us that we were sleep deprived. It basically means creating an environment for yourself that encourages sleep. It includes things such as making the room cooler, using blackout curtains, keeping phones and laptops out of the bedroom, and taking a warm bath or shower before bed (which studies have shown actually help lower body temperature and prepare you for sleep). Some people make journaling or meditation part of their sleep hygiene routine.

But don't forget, your good sleep routine starts earlier in the day. For instance, if you have caffeinated beverages, have them in the morning only—because that 3:00 p.m. pick-me-up can leave you hopped up all the way to 3:00 a.m. And put as much space between dinner, as well as alcoholic beverages, and bedtime as you can. Partially digested food in your GI tract can bother your stomach or give you heartburn, and alcohol can have a drowsy-making effect at bedtime before it wears off and all of a sudden you're wide awake in the middle of the night.

Try Mindful Meditation

Racing thoughts. Recounting bad memories. Reviewing to-do lists. The mind really plays games with us the minute we turn off our bedside lamp. One of the most effective ways to turn off our brain's ticker tape seems to be mindful meditation. This is a type of meditation that focuses on breathing and being in the present while quieting the mind. Many studies, including one from the University of Southern California (USC) and the University of California, Los Angeles (UCLA), suggest that mindfulness meditation can help older adults reduce sleep disturbances and has positive effects on conditions such as depression, stress, and fatigue. Best of all, it's something you can practice in your home, on your own. There are plenty of meditation apps available, even some that cater to menopausal people. I love Insight Timer (www.insighttimer.com) because it has a massive catalog of meditations, teachers, and styles to choose from. And my partner and I use a Tibetan bowl white-noise app to fall asleep every night.

There are also meds specifically prescribed for sleep. They aren't my first-line treatments, as they can cause dependency, diminishing your ability to fall asleep on your own. I typically recommend supplements that enhance the body's natural tendency to sleep. The exception to this is sleep apnea. If you suspect you have sleep apnea—which is when breathing stops and restarts throughout the night—it's probably because your partner said you've been snoring loudly. You may not realize it, but sleep apnea can lead you to get terrible, disrupted sleep. It may also be a sign or precursor of much more serious medical issues, including cardiac disease, stroke, or dementia. To be diagnosed with sleep apnea, you'll have to see a sleep doctor. You may be asked to do a sleep study, where you spend the night in a lab and clinicians track your breathing and other metrics throughout the night. Using that information, you may be prescribed a continuous positive airway pressure (CPAP) machine, which forces air into your nose via a tube. It's quite a contraption and can be intimidating at first, but users report significantly improved sleep almost right away.

Sex and Genitourinary Syndrome of Menopause (GSM) (Yes, We're Talking About It All)

Honestly, I can't believe I'm this far into *Menopause Bootcamp* and we've barely touched upon lube at all. It is *life changing*. And not just during sex. But before I get to that, we need to take a step back and talk about your vagina, vulva, and urinary tract. Take a deep breath, folks. For some participants of the in-person Menopause Bootcamps, this is the point when nervous laughter and squirming in chairs occur. That's because female sex organs—and the subject of sex, itself—become taboo after fifty—which is ridiculous and offensive. You know I'm saddling up my high horse right now about ageism and sexuality, but before I mount, let me put on my doctor coat and give you a bunch of information you need to know.

What Is GSM?

It's a term that was coined in the last several years to encompass several symptoms of menopause that relate to female sexual organs.

Genital symptoms	Vaginal dryness, general discomfort or burning while walking or exercising, irritation, itching, vaginal discharge
Sexual symptoms	Pain during sex, reduction in lubrication, less elasticity in the vaginal canal, lower arousal, reduced or absent orgasm, bleeding after sex
Urinary symptoms	Urinary tract infections, frequency of urination, pain or burning while using the toilet, urinary incontinence

In one multicenter study from Spain—"multicenter" meaning that it was carried out in various institutions—70 percent of menopausal people had GSM and 93.3 percent experienced vaginal dryness. But we are going to change all that. This is one of my favorite topics to talk about in the Menopause Bootcamp because it really changes people's lives. And in talking about it, we start to undo the taboo that befalls GSM and sexuality after menopause. Let's lay it all out there.

The Causes of GSM

The drop in estrogen is the driving force behind GSM. "Estrogen receptors . . . are present in the vagina, vulva, musculature of the pelvic floor, endopelvic fascia"—the connective tissue around the female reproductive organs—"urethra, and bladder trigone," wrote researchers at the Catholic University of Korea in a review published in the *Journal of Menopausal Medicine*. The paper went on to say that the estrogen deficiency that comes with menopause actually alters the female anatomy as well as tissue health. There's a reduction in collagen, hyaluronic acid, and elastin, which causes changes in the pliability of tissues. There are functional changes in smooth muscle cells. The epithelium, a layer of tissue that covers the organs, thins. Connective tissue becomes more dense. And blood vessels disappear. "These changes reduce elasticity of the vagina, increase vaginal pH, lead to changes in vaginal flora, diminish lubrication, and increase vulnerability to physical irritation and trauma."

What Does GSM Feel Like?

Going beyond the chart above, I want to talk about what living with GSM is like. I will go through the symptoms, one by one.

Genital

Dryness is one of the main symptoms of GSM, and I'm not just talking about during sexual arousal. The reason you've been able to walk and run, ride a bike, and do any other physical activity without it paining your vagina and vulva is that your genitals have had natural lubrication. The tissue doesn't get stuck or rub against itself. Take away that natural lubrication, and you've got problems. Chapping and irritation can arise because of this, and since another aspect of GSM is that blood flow is reduced, the body's ability to repair the tissue is diminished. Sometimes irritation can come in the form of itching as well—which is sometimes related to a urinary tract infection. I often liken this to what it would feel like to have constant mouth dryness. Your oral mucosa—lining—is nearly identical to that of the vagina. It is happiest when it's moist and the tissues can easily glide and slide across each other.

How Do I Know if My Vaginal pH Balance Is Off?

A lot of patients ask me about the pH balance of their vagina. I think there's a commercial reason why they're asking: so many products are marketed these days to balance your pH. It's really buzzy. And I have mixed feelings about that. For starters, a general approach to your vagina should be "If it ain't broke, don't fix it." Meaning that unless you're having symptoms of something being wrong, leave your vagina alone. It is a master of cleaning itself and keeping bacteria in check. So vaginal cleaners, odorizers, wipes, and the like are to be avoided. Also, just as an aside, those products are marketed in a really predatory way, making consumers—especially young women—believe that their vaginas are foul smelling and unclean. This contributes to a shame about women's sexuality as something dirty and needing to be managed. I'm not saying that if you see those products on the drugstore shelf, you should shove them to the back behind the tampons, but I'm not saying you shouldn't, either.

However, your vagina is mature now, you know it well, and you may be noticing changes. For instance, during menopause, it may smell different. It's something that your partner may bring up to you. Rest assured, that's not necessarily a warning sign of anything. You may have noticed the same thing during and after pregnancy if you had children. It's indicative of a changing body, and a different chemical balance can change the odor. But you will know if it smells *bad*. That is something to ask your doctor about, as well as reporting itching or discharge, all of which may be indications that the vagina's pH balance is off and there are concomitant microbiome shifts that will favor bacterial strains causing inflammation, leading to discharge or even outright infection. (Microbiomes are areas of microorganisms, like bacteria. Your vagina has a microbiome, as do your GI tract, mouth, and even skin, and they perform a variety of functions. When your microbiome is healthy, your system tends to be healthier, too. If something is off due to illness or imbalance, it throws your system off, too.) A pH balance problem is something your doctor can diagnose, either with a vaginal culture or just by examining the appearance of your vagina.

The vagina likes to live with a pH of 3.8 to 4.5, and that number increases with age. This, in turn, results in a different microbiome and the loss of protective lactobacillus species such as *L. iners* and *L. crispatus*. There are some interesting data demonstrating that the use of boric acid in the vagina to reacidify its pH may help, as can incorporating probiotics or probiotic-promoting food (for instance, yogurt and fermented foods such as kimchi) into your diet and decreasing stress, which can start to undo cortisol-related changes. These could all aid in maintaining a healthy vaginal microbiome.

Your doctor may also recommend a pH-balanced vaginal moisturizer or localized vaginal hormone therapy. There are even some energy devices such as radio-frequency and carbon dioxide lasers that can help restore the tissue changes GSM has caused; you can review them with an experienced clinician.

But don't forget: if you're sexually active, you may have a sexually transmitted infection! Having an evaluation with exam and cultures is key to understanding what is going on, why it is happening, and how to address your particular concerns.

Sexual

For a lot of people, GSM means painful masturbation and penetrative sex, followed possibly by bleeding. When the tissue that makes up the vulva (the external part of the female genitalia) and the vagina (the internal part, also known as the birth canal) experiences GSM, it becomes thinner and more prone to trauma, including bruising and tearing. This probably does not make you want to have penetrative sex! And the longer you go without, the shorter and narrower the vagina becomes, which compounds the issue. Then, when you do have sex, the vulvovaginal tissues, which are less strong and supple than they used to be, are even more prone to injury and pain.

The vagina is often compared to an accordion: When you're young, it has a ton of supple pleats that can expand easily. And during pregnancy, the body is really drenched in estrogen, which is a benefit during labor, since it gives the vaginal canal even more latitude to expand to accommodate the baby's passage. Later in life, though, the pleats start to flatten out so that it's less pliable. And the tissues become drier and more prone to tearing. The less you use the "accordion," the more it breaks down. Basically, it turns into a PVC pipe, as my mentor, Dr. Michael Krychman, a doctor of sexual medicine and gynecologist in southern California, puts it. It's a vicious cycle.

Urinary

There are a couple of aspects to this, the first being pain upon urination. The urethra and bladder are derived from the same type of tissue as the vaginal canal is, so they are subject to the same changes with age and loss of estrogen. Urine itself is quite acidic. Changes to the urinary tract include thinning, more fragile tissue that can be more susceptible to damage, microbiome shifts, inflammation, and infections. Putting delicate, changing tissues into contact with urine may feel worse than before. Often, we feel as though we have a urinary tract infection (UTI) when, in fact, it's merely inflammation—which does not require antibiotic treatments, which would throw off the microbiome even more. But this situation does require an evaluation by your physician and treatment to decrease all of the changes and symptoms. And of course, the problem could very well be a UTI. Decreasing the prevalence of harmful bacteria may assist in prevention; two supplements that might help are D-mannose and cranberry extract, both of which have some data to suggest that they may help and definitely won't harm. "Hygiene products," on the other hand, are really problematic: they shift the bacteria counts in an unhealthy way, and severely increase the risk of vaginal and urinary tract discomfort, inflammation, and infections.

Incontinence is another common issue. It falls into two broad categories: urge incontinence, which is the sudden need to urinate, and stress incontinence, which happens when a sudden movement (such as a sneeze) causes urine to leak. Urge incontinence is related to bladder wall instability, which may become worse for all the same reasons that the urinary tract changes during menopause. But stress incontinence is more related to pelvic floor changes and loss of muscle tone. Stress incontinence can be addressed with pelvic floor exercises and direct application of topical vaginal hormones. Energy devices such as high-intensity focused electromagnetic technology (HIFEM) for pelvic floor contractions and radio-frequency (RF) to increase blood flow, collagen, and elasticity have been shown to decrease both forms of mild to moderate incontinence. They can be expensive, but if they can prevent ongoing or worsening incontinence, that's preferable to surgery—which fails in 30 percent or more of those who undergo it.

The Mind-Body Connection

In the next part of this book, we're going to move on from the biological explanations of menopause and onto how all of this affects us psychologically. But I really have to say one thing at this point about how all of these symptoms of GSM impact us emotionally and how it all gets wrapped up into the larger feelings that we have during and after menopause. Let's take penetrative sex, for example. There's a belief that our sexual desire goes down after menopause. And, like so many aspects of sexuality, this one is . . . complicated.

Sexual desire consists of drive, beliefs, and motivations. Drive or libido is the biological component, including everything from attraction to erotic thoughts and sensations, and it varies greatly from person to person and from day to day. Our belief in our own sexuality is impacted by culture, media, family, and upbringing. Motivation is the most complex, as it is driven by interpersonal relationships and emotional factors.

Although sexual desire can decline with age, women seem to experience a two to three times greater decline in their middle years—although this also varies. Many feel liberated from fears of pregnancy or the need for contraception and experience an increase in libido. About a third of women in the forty-five-to-sixty-four-year-old age range describe having decreased libido, but only 10 percent overall are distressed by the change, and depression and relationship status are factors as well.

Libido changes are not clearly related to one change but are a combinaton of declining estrogen and possibly testosterone levels (the data don't seem to be consistent here), social factors such as stress, mood disorders, and relationship factors or lack of partners, and the discomfort of estrogen loss, sleep disturbances, and other classic menopause symptoms.

But for some, if not most, there's still sexual desire, even if you're not as horny as you were in your twenties. And here's where GSM can get involved. If every time you have penetrative sex or start to masturbate, it hurts and burns and then your vagina is painful for the next week, it is not a huge surprise that the thought of those activities is a turnoff.

Now it feels as if these formerly pleasurable activities are off limits to you. Let's play this out a little: GSM has eroded your desire for intimacy, which now creates a rift between you and your partner. That feels shitty, too. In summation, your dry vagina has changed the relationship you have with yourself and your ability to find sexual pleasure and has thrown a wedge between you and your intimate partner or partners. That's an example of how the psychic stress of menopause manifests itself.

The same can be said for other symptoms. Running used to be liberating, but your vulva's tissue has become so delicate that the activity is painful. You have an opportunity to go on a cool boat trip, but you have to go to the bathroom three times an hour, and making that many trips to the head will be embarrassing, so you decline. Truly, I understand people who say that menopause sucks. The good news is that there are solutions.

Ways to Restore the Vagina

Some say that my adulation of personal lubricant and sexual lube is a little overboard and an indication that I need to find a hobby. You may be right, but give me an opportunity to convert you. Those are two among four broad ways to combat GSM. The other two are vaginal hormonal therapies and energy devices.

Use Personal Moisturizers and Sexual Lubricants

The names give them away: one is to address everyday discomfort, the other is for sexual play, penetrative sex, and masturbation. There are some general principles that apply to both.

1. "All natural" is not always better! Coconut oil is lovely for the skin and may be okay for vulvar dryness and irritation. But it absorbs

rapidly into tissues, so it isn't great for sex. I do recommend some plant-based products, but make sure you're not allergic to them!

2. For everyday activities not related to sex, look for products labeled "personal lubricants or moisturizers." Coconu and Good Clean Love make nice ones. And consider pH-balancing personal lubes such as Luvena Vaginal Moisturizer & Lubricant and Kindra's Vaginal Lotion.

3. Many readily recognized over-the-counter brands really are not the best for sex—if the tissues absorb too much or if fluid is pulled out of them by the product, it results in *more* friction and tissue damage! Silicone-based products are by far the winners. They stay slick, are not absorbed, and usually don't stain your sheets. They are also latex-condom safe. My favorites are Uberlube and Sliquid. Sylk, made from kiwi vine extract, is also good.

4. Remember, even if you can't get pregnant, you can still get a sexually transmitted disease. If you're using condoms to prevent STIs, you cannot use an oil-based lube.

5. Be careful with lube and toys. Read the manufacturers' labels to find out which lubes may be damaging. For example: silicone toy + silicone lube = bad bad bad.

6. Stay away from glycerin, which is drying and irritating. The package may say that it'll be warming, cooling, and all that nonsense. It is mostly going to sting or burn.

7. There is always some trial and error. Preferences differ, as do bodies' responses.

And if you haven't yet tried CBD lube yet, give it a go. CBD is derived from the hemp plant. There are CBD receptors—endocannabinoid receptors—all over your body. The uterus is rich in them. There's a fair amount of research that CBD aids in ovulation and other ovarian and reproductive functions, and there is robust research demonstrating that the body's own endocannabinoid system, which is designed to respond to cannabinoids produced within our bodies, is abundant in tissues associated with sexual function, including the brain, uterus, ovaries, and adrenals, which produce hormones. The confluence of potential relations, pain and pleasure modulation, has tremendous potential in the treatment of sexual dysfunction. For some, CBD may help reduce sexual pain associated with menopausal changes to the vaginal and vulvar region, allow muscles to relax, which helps with pliability, and act as a libido enhancer.

But let's be honest: Did you ever smoke a doobie in college and get horny? Welp! There you go! This makes me really excited (pun?) to recommend cannabis-infused lubes and suppositories to those who are noticing declining response, enjoyment, and interest in sex and masturbation. The clinical research is just starting to emerge, but it's promising, and trying this approach is low risk.

Use Vaginal Hormone Therapy

This is a huge topic, but priming the pump—restoring blood flow and protecting the mucosa—goes a long way toward restoring your sexual organs' ability to get or stay lubricated. But if you've delayed using any lube, or your vagina for that matter, for years or if you have more stubborn discomfort, blood flow may be compromised and this may take a while to restore. And a quick note about safety: Contrary to popularly held beliefs, *they are not absorbed into your body and are safe for everyone.* They cannot affect clotting, strokes, heart disease, or cancer!

Use Energy Devices

This is an underused treatment that can be really effective. Administered in a medical setting, these devices cause microdamage to the vaginal tissue. That microdamage causes an inflammatory response, and because of it, a regrowth of blood vessels and collagen occurs and tissue health is restored. This effect can last six months to a year after the procedure is complete. Energy devices work best in synergy with vaginal hormone therapy. The problem? It's expensive and not covered by insurance. Can I just say: It's wild to me that so many people need to pay out of pocket for menopause-related meds and procedures. This is life-changing stuff.

Use Vaginal Estrogen Therapy

If the cause of GSM is the reduction in circulating estrogen, it stands to reason that estrogen replacement can help. And some women do opt to do hormone treatments postmenopause—and GSM is one of the factors that plays into that decision. However, vaginal estrogen therapy is a more direct way to treat GSM using much less estrogen. You'll begin to notice a difference quite soon after starting. The vaginal hormone therapy I most often prescribe to my patients is DHEA or prasterone, which is a precursor hormone. Once you insert it into your vagina (as a capsule, tablet, ring, or cream), it's absorbed into the vaginal tissue. The DHEA is then converted by your body's enzymes into whatever your system needs and wants—either testosterone or estrogen.

Precursor hormones: What are they? You know the ongoing debate around stem cells and their use in research? The reason they're coveted in science is because embryonic cells—the ones that make up frozen embryos for in vitro fertilization—end up differentiating and becoming all of the cells throughout the body. Various chemical signals tell stem cells to become bone cells, liver cells, or upper lip skin cells. If a growing embryo is like a building under construction, those chemical signals are the construction foreman that tells each cell where it should go and what it should become.

That's the same basic idea behind precursor hormones. They are more basic, yet actualized, hormones that have the potential to become different things. DHEA, for example, can become either estrogen or testosterone. And the body has hormone receptors that, when they come in contact with the DHEA, use it for what they need. That helps explain why DHEA may be safer for some patients than, say, oral hormone replacement treatment. Rather than suffusing the body with estrogen, the DHEA, when placed in the vagina, disperses a little of this precursor hormone, which is utilized only by the genital tissue that needs a bump.

The good news is that there's strong research suggesting that it's safe to use in just about everybody—including cancer patients or survivors who can't take hormone replacement therapy.

Vaginal estrogen therapy comes in four forms:

1. **Cream.** Using an applicator, you'll insert this into your vagina every day for one to three weeks at first, and then the frequency will taper off per your doctor's instructions. It can get a little messy, so most people choose to do this at night. But it's also great for soothing more external parts such as the vulva, the entrance (or introitus) where penetration most often feels uncomfortable, and around the clitoris and urethra.

2. **Suppositories.** Similarly to the cream, these capsules are inserted into the vagina every day for a few weeks; then your doctor will tell you when to switch to twice a week. Again, most women wait to use it at bedtime.

3. **Ring.** Like its birth control cousin, this flexible ring is placed in the vagina and slowly releases estrogen. You place it yourself and replace it every three months.

4. **Tablet.** A tablet goes directly into the vagina via an applicator and dissolves. Usually, you place it every day for a couple weeks before switching to twice a week according to a schedule your doctor will give you that is tailored for you.

Vaginal Estrogen Therapy and Cancer

A lot of you will have rightfully been told by your doctor that hormone replacement therapy isn't in the cards for you due to the cancer risk. This specifically applies to people who have been diagnosed with a hormone-sensitive cancer, particularly breast cancer, or have a strong family history of cancer. However, according to the American College of Obstetricians and Gynecologists (ACOG), the data say that women who have a history of breast cancer or are undergoing treatment don't have an increased risk of recurrence if they use vaginal estrogen for GSM symptoms. This is because the estrogen contained seems to remain in the vagina rather than entering the bloodstream and circulating throughout the body. Therefore, the risk of the low-dose estrogen "feeding" any microscopic cancer in the body is, according to the research, essentially zero.

That being said, the ACOG does recommend that people try nonhormonal therapies first and, if those don't work, move on to low-dose vaginal estrogen. This is a pretty common approach in ob-gyn: basically, we are fairly certain that it will be totally fine, but out of an abundance of caution, let's use it as a last resort. I'm fine with that approach, generally speaking. There are patients of mine, though, who have such awful GSM symptoms that are really ruining their lives, and for them I may go ahead and recommend low-dose vaginal estrogen right off the bat.

Eat Healthy Fats

Your vagina wants you to eat avocado toast for breakfast and whole wheat pasta with glugs of olive oil for dinner. Avocado and extra-virgin olive oil are forms of healthy fats that, along with fatty fish such as sardines and salmon, as well as nuts, are the basis of the body's natural production of DHEA. (Lack of fat intake partially explains why women who suffer from anorexia lose their periods; their body's estrogen level is too low.)

Get Your Blood Pumping

You'll hear me talk about working out a lot, because it's one of the closest remedies we have to a silver bullet. Truly, getting your blood pumping with cardio will increase blood flow to your genitals, which helps keep the cell tissues healthy and turning over. It also keeps you flexible, which is great for masturbation and partnered sex play—which is great for the tissues, too. Weight lifting and strength work will also help your pelvic floor, which will combat incontinence as well as improve sex. And all those endorphins—feel-good hormones—that are released during exercise help you feel more sexy and powerful, which you can use as you deal with GSM.

The Moral of the Vagina Story: Use It or Lose It

If you have unaddressed GSM symptoms, they will get worse with time. They will negatively affect your day-to-day life and your sex life. Get proactive about GSM. Try out different moisturizers and lubes. Get reacquainted with masturbation if it's been a little while. If you can afford an energy device treatment, try it; I've never had a patient who thought it wasn't worth it, myself included.

Weight Gain (If You Think I'm Going to Give You a Magic Diet, You're Reading the Wrong Book)

For a lot of people, this is a tough part of menopause, so I'm going to approach it in a few ways: medically, emotionally, and socially. A disclaimer here: I've personally struggled with weight gain. Well, gaining the weight wasn't a struggle; losing it was. And then, while researching this book and learning that some of my beliefs about the unhealthiness of living in a bigger body weren't all medically accurate—that was a struggle. And then pairing that new knowledge with my experience of being a woman in the world and living in Los Angeles, well, yeah, I continue to ride the Struggle Bus on this issue. But if I'm a passenger, I imagine that some of you are, too. This is too big of a topic to tackle in one section—after all, whole books have been written about it—so we're going to start with an explanation as to why you're prone to gaining weight and the medical evidence as to why it may be something to worry about. Or not worry, as more literature suggests.

Talking about weight from the perspective of a physician is tricky. The idea of an ideal weight is actually not straightforward in the medical literature, although we do know that some diseases, such as heart disease and cancer, are associated with obesity. For those who are concerned about weight management, I classify weight loss as part of self-care and overall good health, and I'm challenging myself and you to separate health and appearance. But I'm going to kick that can down the road for the moment and do a quick lecture on the biology of menopause-related weight gain.

Metabolism, Meet Menopause

There's a common perception that metabolism slows down during menopause and that's why the life change brings added weight. And it is true that hormonal changes can affect metabolism. But there are

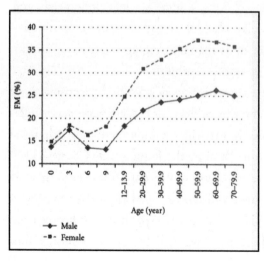

FIGURE 1
Percentage of fat mass (FM) in males and females showing the divergence that occurs at puberty and persists through the premenopausal years.

a couple things to keep in mind. One, believe it or not, is that our percentage of fat mass steadily increases over our lifetime, starting with puberty and going throughout our premenopausal years, according to Australian researchers. That's true for both men and women. That's something to keep in mind.

Maybe I need to take a step back and explain metabolism. At its most basic, metabolism is the process of turning fuel into energy. For humans, that fuel is what we eat and drink, and the energy supports our organ functions. I want to stop for a second and double down on that last point: most of what we consume is used by the body to keep all of its parts going. The brain uses a ton of fuel, and its preferred source is carbohydrates. For the lungs to draw in air and expel carbon dioxide, for the heart to pump life-giving oxygenated blood to every cell, for the GI tract to keep doing its thing, not to mention the kidneys and liver, energy is needed to maintain the system. And that's when you're at rest. Even more energy is needed to, like, do stuff.

The energy needs of the body and the rate at which the body turns fuel into energy are separate but related. Energy needs, which boil down to the amount of calories and macronutrients—fats, carbohydrates, and protein—a person requires to keep the system running in top form are individualized. Muscle increases metabolic needs, too. And, of course, genetics play a big role in overall body composition— probably the greatest role, more than upbringing and lifestyle—which in turn influences your metabolic attributes.

How this all happens is not settled science. We're still learning about how metabolism works and what influences it. Case in point: In 2021, the journal *Science* caused a stir when it published an article titled "Daily Energy Expenditure Through the Human Life Course." Dozens of international researchers assembled data from more than six thousand people, both male and female, aged eight days to ninety-five years, to understand the total energy expenditure of people from birth to old age. What they found was that energy expenditure jumps up in the first year of life and through childhood, then declines by 3 percent per year until we're in our early twenties. It's then that energy expenditure plateaus, and then, at age sixty, it begins to decline again, at a rate of 0.7 percent per year. Loss of muscle mass is part of the reason for the later-in-life slowdown, as is cellular aging; as we get older, cellular turnover in all parts of our bodies takes longer.

I understand that this discussion can be triggering for some people. Considering that we're drowning in diet culture, it is conceivable that it's at least a little triggering for *everybody*. I want to relay this information neutrally, so we are all starting this conversation from the same place. Our metabolism is a reflection of, among other things, the amount of energy our body expends growing, repairing, carrying out its normal bodily functions such as keeping our heart beating and our brain thinking, and doing all of our physical activities on top of that: frolicking on the beach, running after a bus, writing to our congressperson demanding that he or she vote for body autonomy. Fat is a form of energy that the body stores for later usage. It is also the body's backup plan in case food is scarce and has a protective function for certain organs. For instance, did you know that there's an organ in the body called the omentum? It's situated over the abdomen and protects the liver, intestines, and stomach. And there's the possibly apocryphal story zooming around the internet that women's abdomens— especially the area below the belly button—have fat stored there to protect (or possibly feed) their internal organs. I did some sleuthing and couldn't find anything definitive, but it's helpful to think about stored fat in a positive light.

Metabolic Changes and Body Image

When I started to put pen to paper, the issue of how our bodies change as we move into this stage was front and center. It is one of the most common and thorny concerns that face us and that you bring to me, your doctor. I so want to help you, to help us all, reconcile how we feel, how we look, and what is actually healthy to do. I have been honest over the years with my own patients about how difficult it has been for me to address the concerns of the flabby belly, the thickening midsection, the inability to keep your weight where you want it while doing nothing different in your life—same amount of exercise, same diet. In reading, researching, and talking to the experts and doing my own (forgive the double entendre) gut check, I came to a few conclusions—some of which you may not love because I know you may be wishing that I'm about to deliver the magic bullet.

My social media feeds are *full* of ads for tips and tricks to lose belly fat. My feeds are also full of experts in integrative medicine and nutrition proclaiming the next superfood to cure slowing metabolism. I see a trend of otherwise healthy, slim humans wearing continuous glucose monitors, which are designed for diabetics to monitor blood sugars and help keep them alive, purportedly to track their insulin resistance and manage their weight. It's head-spinningly confusing and overwhelming.

Even as I planned this section of the book, I felt inadequate to review this huge topic for you because of my own disordered relationship with food and eating. When I have taught this section of the Menopause Bootcamp, I have called it "Weight and Metabolism," and only recently did I realize what it means to a patient to call it that and how very wrongheaded it is.

Hear me out.

According to large population studies such as the CDC's National Health and Nutrition Examination Survey (NHANES), the percentage of American women who are considered "overweight" or "affected by obesity" increases from 51.7 percent to 68.1 percent during midlife. The average weight gain at the time of the menopausal transition is five pounds, with about 20 percent of women in the United States gaining ten pounds or more.

We do understand the physiology of these changes, some of which are not unique to women and are merely consequences of aging. Dr. Melina Jampolis, an internist and board-certified physician nutrition specialist, reminded me that our estrogen level declines, our androgens increase, we lose lean body mass, and consequently our insulin resistance increases. Our sleep duration and quality decline. Our mood fluctuates, as does our cortisol level. The hormones that control appetite and satiety—leptin and ghrelin—are impacted. Belly fat is deposited in response to this, and of course I think we all know that so-called truncal obesity contributes to metabolic syndrome and the risk of developing cardiac disease, diabetes, stroke, and cancer.

Talking to the menopause nutrition expert Jenn Salib Huber, RD, ND, was eye opening. She shared with me the story of discovering an unknown half sister in her forties and finding a woman who had been raised in a totally different environment whose body looks *exactly like hers.* She shared that she can buy clothes sight unseen for herself based merely on her sister's fit. It turns out that 70 to 80 percent of body type and composition are determined by genetics, and Jenn's experience is just one example of this powerful influence. We do know that epigenetics are powerful mitigators of our fixed DNA sequences. According to Dr. Jampolis, our activity level (sorry, a gentle thirty-minute stroll won't do it unless you have until now been 100 percent couch potatoing it) and the development and maintenance of lean body mass (i.e., increasing our muscle mass via weight-bearing exercise) are things we can impact and probably don't do enough of. There are also supplements and lifestyle changes we will discuss later on that can decrease our insulin resistance (making us more efficient users of both carbohydrates and fat) and thus rev up our metabolism to make it a more efficient burner of fuel—i.e., food.

This poses the question: Which is more powerful—genetics or lifestyle—and how hard do we need to work to make changes? How hard do we want to work? Will what we do be effective? And what is the driving motivation for this change? It is borderline impossible to distinguish our own desire for a long, healthy life from the influences of the patriarchy and diet culture. We still associate being thin with being healthy, and a slim body is still overwhelmingly considered to be the beauty standard. At the very least, if you are reading this book, you were probably raised in a time when Cheryl Tiegs and Farrah Fawcett were the ideal beauties: tall, slim, blond. You cannot tell me that those images didn't imprint themselves on your young spongelike brain and negatively impact your perceptions of health and beauty. I was raised in a home where food was an obsession. My parents were *constantly* dieting, and body size was a regular source of concern, shame, and conflict. I struggle to this day with remembering that my body is a vehicle and a means of experiencing this life and is, in and of itself, a blessing.

As the body positivity movement has gained momentum, I have also seen a quiet backlash in the medical community of "but obesity!" Although a certain amount of fatness does increase the risk of developing serious health issues, self-acceptance must be a part of menopause in general and weight specifically. If we can focus on the psychological and spiritual aspects of feeling happy and at home in our bodies, even as they change, I think we can face the challenges of aging most effectively. This requires a capacity to accept changes that we may not like, grieve what we have lost or maybe never even had, and embrace what is and what can be. This is what is called embodiment. In plain-ish English, "Embodiment theory—that we use our own bodily experience and processes to understand our own emotional experience, and the experiences of others—has provided a mechanism to help us understand emotional processing."

The presence of fat, in and of itself, does not tell you much about the overall health of a person. Read that again: *The presence of fat, in and of itself, does not tell you much about the overall health of a person.* If you find that hard to believe, that's okay. A few years ago, I'm not sure I would've written that, either. The caveat is, of course, that body sizes sit along a spectrum, and a person with a body that's much too small to be healthy and functional is somewhat identifiable, and someone who is much too large to be healthy and functional is somewhat identifiable. But if you just give me a person's body mass index (BMI) score, which is a representation of the relationship of their weight to their height, for 99 percent of people, there is zero usable information in it. For instance, you can tell me that someone is in the healthy range for BMI, but it turns out that their cholesterol levels are off the charts. Similarly, someone can be in the obese range, yet all of their markers for blood sugar, cholesterol, resting heart rate, and more are perfectly fine. That's why weight is a red herring—and one that doctors and society have been dangerously obsessed with for the past several decades.

Still, I don't want to entirely discount the theory that excess fat can be a warning sign of or contribute to developing diseases such as cancer, heart disease, hypertension, type 2 diabetes, gallbladder disease, stroke risk, and joint problems—which happen to be diseases associated with the menopause transition. But I think it's fair to say that fat is pretty much never the sole cause of any of these diseases. Things such as a person's diet, exercise habits, smoking and drinking status, lifelong or current exposure to pollution, existence of a support system, and genetics all play a bigger role in whether a person will develop disease than does the existence of fat alone.

My patients, I think, want me to tell them how to lose weight, and not just to commiserate with them about how hard it is. Because it is really, really hard. What's more, most people who lose weight gain it back and then some. When I think about the long-term changes I want my patients to make in order to live long, healthy lives, weight loss isn't the be-all and end-all. In fact, a focus on weight loss might be detrimental for many of them. And losing weight is the advice of far too many doctors. There are so many horror stories of women going to their doctors with a variety of symptoms, such as pain, fatigue, or general off-ness; the doctor takes one look at them, tells them to lose weight, and sends them on their way. Meanwhile, the woman has cancer or an autoimmune disorder, and the dismissive doctor could only see her weight. To make matters worse, that woman probably now feels really shitty and is unlikely to go get a second opinion. If you think I'm overstating this, consider a questionnaire generated by researchers at the University of Pennsylvania, the findings of which were published in a paper titled "Primary Care Physicians' Attitudes About Obesity and Its Treatment." The study found that over half of physicians viewed obese patients as "awkward, unattractive, ugly, and noncompliant." It was published in 2003, but I don't think that medical training and overall mindsets have changed enough to call into question the consistency of those responses or whether those beliefs are still held today.

I don't want to get too much in the weeds about this just yet. Let's circle back to menopause. Yes, it's not surprising if you gain weight. Yes, I support you if you want to work on your eating, exercise, and stress reduction habits in healthy ways and if the net effect of those efforts is to maintain your premenopausal weight or to reduce if you gained weight. But a small yet growing cadre of doctors is more concerned with metrics other than weight. Now, I'm not a general practitioner, so your GP will be the one who attends to some of the metrics I've listed below. But as part of your health care team, I'll certainly keep an eye on them. Some data will be specific to you and your family history, but the universal ones include:

Your vitamin D3 level. We know that calcium is necessary for strong bones, but vitamin D helps bones absorb and use that calcium. And estrogen helps activate vitamin D. The loss of estrogen means that the body isn't using vitamin D efficiently. Plus, research has found that this vitamin plays a crucial role in reducing inflammation by regulating the body's production of immune cells and inflammatory cytokines. And we know that inflammation is a huge risk factor for major medical illnesses associated with aging, such as cancer. Vitamin D is made by the body when you're exposed to the sun, but your doctor may see that you have an insufficiency and put you on a supplement.

Inflammatory markers. There are a few of them, but research is starting to coalesce around measuring C-reactive protein (CRP) to rule out diseases and detect infections, autoimmune diseases, and cancers.

Your hemoglobin A1C level. This single test measures your average blood sugar level during the past few months and can help diagnose type 1 and type 2 diabetes. A high A1C level means that your blood sugar isn't under control and you are at risk of developing diabetes (or have uncontrolled diabetes). This test is crucial if you ever had gestational diabetes.

Your blood pressure. Recently, the guidelines for what is a healthy blood pressure have changed. And if you have a history of pregnancy-related blood pressure issues, this is critical to stay on top of because we know that pregnancy is "the ultimate stress test," according to Dr. Suzanne Steinbaum, a holistic cardiologist, the onetime director of women's cardiovascular prevention, health and wellness at Mount Sinai Hospital in New York City, president of the lifestyle management program SRSHeart, and author of *Dr. Suzanne Steinbaum's Heart Book: Every Woman's Guide to a Heart-Healthy Life.*

Your cholesterol levels. Getting a yearly fasting lipid test can help monitor changes in the types of cholesterol and their ratios to each other. These are important markers of cardio-metabolic status.

Your resting heart rate. The menopausal transition can reveal underlying heart issues, including transient arrhythmias, or more serious problems, such as metabolic disorder.

Your heart rate variability. This more sensitive assessment of heart health measures the severity of menopausal symptoms such as hot flashes, which may actually be early signs of heart disease

---

Frequently Asked Question:
Should I Take a Women's Supplement?

If we're talking about random over-the-counter women's vitamins, the answer is meh, probably not. The problem is that although they're marketed to people in your age group who are postmenopausal, they're not tailored to your specific needs. The types of multivitamins I so often see usually try to cram so much stuff in one pill that it's not really giving you enough of any one thing. Think of it as being like a cookie: if you add chocolate chips, walnuts, coconut, dried cranberries, and flaxseed to the batter, that cookie is going to get really big and bulky. Well, it's the same with a vitamin supplement: the more you cram into it, the less you get of each thing. This is also done for consumers' benefit; vitamin manufacturers don't know if you are eating a fairly well-balanced diet and need some help with a few specific vitamins or if you live in a food desert where fresh produce is hard to come by and you need a supplement to give you a lot of the basics that your diet can't provide. Overdosing on vitamins is possible and is not a great thing. So vitamin makers play it safe.

Now, that does not mean that vitamin and mineral supplements aren't helpful. They are, as long as they're tailored to your diet and your body's needs. Your doctor can talk with you about your diet and other lifestyle factors, and you may decide together that you would benefit from a specific vitamin or supplement or a combination of them; sometimes you get the most out of a certain supplement when it's taken along with something else, such as vitamin D3 with K2 or calcium with magnesium. Or maybe the problem isn't having enough of a certain substance; rather, it's the lack of a helper substance.

The Power of Many

I feel the need to take a moment to remind all of us that Menopause Bootcamp works not only because it's straight talk about what's happening to your body but also because it creates a community of women who support one another. This is not a nice-to-have—it's a need-to-have. I hope that when you read about hot flashes, vaginal dryness, and weight gain, you pictured all of the other people who were in the same boat as you. We just don't *talk* about this shit. When people ask how we're doing, we say "Great!" with a chirpiness that dissuades follow-up questions.

But I know that this experience can be really emotional. I see it in my patients' eyes when we're having these big conversations. And I worry sometimes about what kind of support systems they have to go home to, particularly the older women. My worry is certainly justified. Loneliness has become an epidemic in this country. According to testimony before the Senate, one in five Americans say they feel lonely or isolated, which some experts say is as harmful as smoking fifteen cigarettes a day. That's a serious number, and it means we have a serious problem. Part of it is cultural. We live in a society in which families don't necessarily stay together, and menopause occurs around the time a woman's children, if she has them, are leaving the nest to start lives of their own. Which all means that it can be a vulnerable— and lonely—time for many women.

That's part of why I created the Menopause Bootcamp. All of us, together, seek to tap into the power of community to help ourselves— and one another. This isn't just a warm and fuzzy talking point; there is a growing body of research showing that health outcomes improve when people are part of a community. That's true whether a group forms out of necessity—to help people overcome addiction, adopt and maintain healthy habits, or manage their diabetes—or focuses on general well-being, such as controlling stress and other factors that influence health. Even if it's just an informal group of friends, finding a community of people with whom you can talk about menopause makes a difference. I wanted to tell you this in case you were feeling overwhelmed by all the information I'm throwing at you. So deep breaths all together, and let's keep going.

Changes in Hair, Skin, Teeth, and Nails
(Hey, Older Generation: A Heads-up
About Them Would've Been Nice)

Our old hormone friend estrogen is behind these changes, too. In the same way as its presence makes the genitals strong, pliable, and hydrated, estrogen has an effect on skin. After you have the first symptoms of menopause—say, hot flashes and night sweats or GSM—you may start to notice that your skin looks thinner, a few more wrinkles show up that you hadn't noticed before, you have to put on lotion more often due to dryness, and overall, your skin has lost its elasticity. Those are some of the characteristics outlined in a paper by researchers at the University of Bradford in 2007. You may also notice that your hair loses its luster and breaks more easily than it used to. Your nails are less strong. You may need more dental work. All of this is menopause related.

It seems that estrogen plays a role in the body's collagen production. Collagen is a protein. In fact, it's the most abundant protein in the body. It's a building block of bones, tendons, ligaments, skin, hair, eyes, teeth, and nails. Collagen gets a boost from estrogen, so you can imagine what happens when that hormone wanes. Estrogen is also a really important factor in good blood circulation. When it drops off, the skin gets less moisture and loses elasticity.

Each person's skin and hair needs are individualized and based on things such as genetics, inflammatory skin conditions such as psoriasis that may worsen during menopause, history of sun exposure, and experiences with certain prescription drugs and treatments such as chemotherapy. But there are a few things you can do to help the situation.

Hydrate Your Skin

One reason your skin feels drier is that because of the drop in estrogen and collagen levels, it retains less water. Blood and lymphatic fluid flow is less robust, too, so you're not getting as much natural moisturization and cell turnover is slowed. According to the American Academy of Dermatology, you can adjust your skin care routine to address your symptoms. Use a mild cleanser to wash your skin, and apply moisturizers that contain hyaluronic acid or glycerin as needed—rosewater with glycerin is a favorite! Applying a moisturizer to damp (not wet) skin makes a huge difference in retaining hydration. Oil-based products are also wonderful lubricating options, particularly if you have dry skin. Other things to do:

♦ Exfoliate sparingly. Yes, back in the day, we scrubbed down with the most abrasive exfoliants we could find. But since menopause makes the skin thinner, too much roughing up can cause damage and redness that don't repair themselves as fast as before.

♦ If the skin on your body becomes itchy or uncomfortable, use a cool compress on the affected part, or take a cool bath with colloidal oatmeal—finely ground oatmeal—which has anti-inflammatory properties.

♦ If you're experiencing acne due to changing hormones, use a cleanser with benzoyl peroxide, and spot treat with an adapalene gel—but avoid acne reducers that contain salicylic acid, which doesn't work the same way on mature skin as it does on teenage skin.

◆ *Of course* you're already slathering on a broad-spectrum sunscreen when you go outside, right? Sun protection may help fade age spots and stop new ones from forming. One constant among my patients with the healthiest-looking visages: they apply a facial moisturizer with SPF every morning.

◆ Drink enough water. That advice is going to come up often. Also, be aware that alcohol is a dehydrator that affects your skin. Cigarettes, e-cigarettes, and vape pens are bad—not only for your skin but also for the rest of you. (I know you know that, but I'm a doctor and I can't help it.) A diet laden with antioxidant-rich produce, healthy fats, and lean protein will keep your body's largest organ—the skin—feeling and looking good.

Pay Your Dermatologist an Annual Visit

Skin cancer is by far the most frequently diagnosed type of cancer, and in your menopausal years is a prime time to develop it. The reason skin cancer can show up now is that years of exposure to the sun and other toxins have laid the groundwork for malignancies, combined with the fact that your skin cells are not turning over as quickly as they once did. Do skin checks every couple weeks when you shower, and tell your dermatologist about any changes or spots you've discovered. They will also do a skin check. Additionally, a cosmetic dermatologist can fill you in on the latest topical medications, treatments, and procedures that might be right for you if you want to restore your skin's elasticity or glow. Those treatments can cost hundreds or even thousands of dollars and aren't covered by insurance. It's a personal choice if they're something you want to explore.

One Don't: *Don't Use Menopausal Hormone Therapy for Skin Issues*

Yes, it's logical to think that hormone replacement therapy will help rehydrate your skin and boost your collagen level. And for some people, it does. However, this shouldn't be the driving force behind your decision to take MHT. In all honesty, it probably won't work very well unless treatment is initiated well before the menopausal transition is over.

Bone Health (Take Care of Your Bones, and They'll Take Care of You)

I know what you're thinking. I've hit you with dry vagina, less elastic skin, and now we're moving right along to weak bones. I can't really sugarcoat it because these are all things that are happening. But they are (a) not a death sentence; (b) not a judgment on you, your personal agency, or your potential; and (c) all things that we can ameliorate with behavior changes and some over-the-counter supplements and aids. Take a deep breath, because we're now going to talk about the other Big O: osteoporosis.

What Is Osteoporosis?

This is a condition in which the bones deteriorate, the body doesn't make enough bone to replace the bone lost, or both. When you're in your twenties, your bones are dense, but they're not solid. Instead, they have a honeycomb pattern. Just like the rest of your body, bone is made up of cells that your body has to "keep up"; resorption is when the bones get rid of old cells, and ossification is when they make new ones. This also happens when a bone is fractured; the damaged bone cells need to get cleaned up, and new ones need to be made to fix the break. Young, healthy people have bones that are durable because they're dense and mend fairly quickly if they're broken.

This isn't the case for a person with osteoporosis. The bones are less dense, which essentially means that the spaces in the honeycomb are larger. And so if your bones experience a trauma—usually due to a fall—they're more apt to break. And it takes longer for the break to heal. About half of women aged fifty or older will break a bone because of osteoporosis. The danger that comes with a broken bone increases as a person gets older. If breakage happens to vertebrae, the person may suffer from permanent spine damage. A break to a limb can bring limited mobility, and the bone may never quite heal.

How Is Osteoporosis Diagnosed?

An endocrinologist specializes in hormone disorders, and since estrogen loss drives bone issues, that's the specialist you may be referred to. You might also end up visiting a rheumatologist, who is knowledgeable about age-related bone loss. Since osteoporosis is painless, people may not know they're experiencing it until they have a break. But there are diagnostic tools to measure how healthy our skeletons are. Bone density scans, or bone mass measurement tests, are used to determine bone health as well as osteoporosis. Usually they're done with a specialized X-ray machine, but technicians may also do a certain kind of ultrasound or computed tomography (CT). You're given a T-score, which tells you and your doctor if you have normal bone density, low bone density (also called osteopenia), or osteoporosis. If you meet certain risk factors for osteoporosis—if you're over sixty-five, have a family history of osteoporosis, experience a break, or notice bad pain or height loss—your doctor should send you for a bone density scan. It's quick and painless and is almost always covered by insurance (Medicare covers one test every two years).

The Causes of Osteoporosis

We can place a lot of the blame for osteoporosis on the loss of estrogen. Bone cells have estrogen receptors on them, meaning they are "turned on" by the hormone. The loss of estrogen during menopause means that bone metabolism—the process of resorption and ossification—slows down. But that's not the only cause. Vitamin D helps with calcium absorption, so too little of this fat-soluble vitamin—meaning that it needs to be in the presence of fat to break down, as opposed to a water-soluble vitamin such as vitamin C—can cause bones not to utilize calcium properly. Sunlight is a big source of vitamin D, as are fatty fish and egg yolks; some foods, including orange juice and cereal, are fortified with vitamin D as well. So if you're lacking any of these for many years, you may be at risk for less bone density later in life.

While we're on the subject, I highly recommend magnesium for most of my patients. It works synergistically with calcium and vitamin D, meaning that the efficacy of each is aided by the presence of the others. Magnesium is essential for cellular functions that impact bones, muscle, gut, and sleep. Adequate amounts of the mineral may help stave off conditions including migraines, metabolic syndrome, PMS, and cardiac arrhythmias; troublingly, up to two-thirds of people in the Western world don't get enough magnesium, Canadian researchers found. The recommended daily allowance for women is 310 to 320 milligrams per day and for men 400 to 420 milligrams per day. I recommend that magnesium be taken in its taurate or glycinate forms; it can also be found in foods such as pumpkin seeds, almonds, black beans, dark chocolate, peanuts, avocado, and spinach.

Thyroid issues can make you a candidate for osteoporosis. If you have a history of eating disorders, have had low calcium intake for a long time, or have undergone gastric bypass surgery, you are at a higher risk of developing them. And according to the Mayo Clinic, certain medications, including steroids, that are prescribed for certain diseases, including celiac disease, inflammatory bowel disease, kidney and liver disease, cancer, lupus, multiple myeloma, and rheumatoid arthritis, could contribute to osteoporosis later.

How to Improve Your Bone Health

Bones are slow growing, which is a double-edged sword. On the one hand, if you follow good bone health practices, you have a better chance at holding on to your bone density. However, if you have osteoporosis, it's really hard to reverse it. Here's a rundown based on your risk factors.

Good for Everyone

It's pretty standard fare for menopausal people to take a calcium supplement that contains vitamin D. Doing weight-bearing exercises, such as walking or jogging, as well as weight lifting, also helps retain and improve bone density. But before starting either of these, double-check with your doctor. Of course, a healthy diet that's low in processed foods and bursting with colorful produce, healthy fats, and the right mix of carbs and protein can help as well.

Prescribed for Those at Risk of Fractures

Bisphosphonates. There's a class of drugs called bisphosphonates that are usually taken in pill form weekly or monthly but can be given intravenously. Bisphosphonates slow bones from losing calcium and other minerals, and they also pump the brakes on resorption—the process by which older bone cells are cleaned out. That gives the ossification process (making new bone) a chance to catch up, thus slowing the rate of osteoporosis and reducing the chances of a break. Bisphos-phonates come in a few forms:

Alendronate (Binosto, Fosamax)
Etidronate (Didronel)
Ibandronate (Boniva)
Pamidronate (Aredia)
Risedronate (Actonel, Atelvia)
Zoledronic acid (Reclast, Zometa)

They come with sometimes serious side effects, so make sure you understand everything they entail before starting them.

Monoclonal antibodies. You may remember these from the covid-19 pandemic, when older folks diagnosed with the coronavirus received them. Simply put, they are lab-made copies of white blood cells that teach your immune system how to function in a certain way. In the case of covid-19, the monoclonal antibodies taught people's immune systems how to fight off the virus. In people with osteoporosis or a risk for bone breaks, Denosumab slows the breakdown of bone. It's given via injection twice a year, but once you start on it, you may have to continue it indefinitely.

Estrogen-related treatment. There's a drug called raloxifene, marketed under the brand name Evista, that mimics estrogen without creating many of the complications of hormone replacement therapy—though it won't treat hot flashes, and you may find yourself flashing more on the drug. Raloxifene is also prescribed to women who have a risk of invasive breast cancer. It's a pill that's taken daily.

Other drugs. Other drugs are available, some of them more powerful, to treat bone loss. It's important to note that one of the only serious medical conditions that menopausal hormone therapy actually slows or prevents is osteoporosis—though even so, I would not recommend MHT if osteoporosis is the only thing you're trying to treat.

Muscles and Joints (Get Pumped!)

I'm going to address these together because muscles and joints play off each other. The muscles do the moving, and the joints are what moves. When muscles are at their best, they take the brunt of the pressure that movement puts on the body. When joints are at their best, they are lubricated and move easily, allowing body movements to flow. And when one of them starts to degrade, it puts greater pressure on the other. For instance, joint pain can be caused by weakening muscles. And muscle pain can be caused by overcompensation due to a joint problem.

When you reach menopause, muscle and joint issues can crop up. There are two reasons for this, and one of them is hormonal. Estrogen plays an important role in muscle and connective tissue development and retention, so the loss of estrogen has some predictable impacts on muscle. The decline in muscle mass is called *sarcopenia*. The second part is that you've been using your body for decades, and age as well as previous injuries can start to wear down the parts.

Muscle and Menopause

I discussed earlier how our metabolism takes a hit during menopause. One of the reasons is that there is a sharp decline in muscle mass because of the loss of estrogen. The physiological explanation is a little complicated and scientists are still trying to understand it fully, but I'll give you some of the highlights. As we age, our body doesn't utilize protein as efficiently as it did before, while oxidative stress—so-called metabolic waste, the leftover unusable products of your cells' work—and inflammation impair the healthy functioning of muscle tissue, according to a review of research published in the *Journal of Musculoskeletal and Neuronal Interactions*.

These phenomena are true for both women and men. However, menopause seems to exacerbate them. The way the body stores fat changes, too. Human bodies store a certain amount of fat within muscle, and women store more of it. It's a useful reminder that to the body, fat is a fuel source, so storing intramuscular fat is a way for the muscles to tap into fuel when they need to. The body is constantly engaged in a balancing act of storing the right amount of fuel and building the right amount of muscle. This balance gets thrown out of whack during menopause. The body increases the amount of fat actually stored within muscle, but it loses its ability to use it effectively. The balance between muscle and intramuscular fat changes in unhealthy ways.

Meanwhile, the body uses the abdominal region for fat storage. This has several consequences: the ratio of muscle to fat changes, and because of that, insulin sensitivity—the body's ability to metabolize sugar as opposed to storing it as fat—decreases. Also, muscle uses more energy than fat, so a person with a higher muscle mass has a higher metabolism. As menopause eats away at muscle tissue, that helps explain why the rate of metabolism is on the decline, too. Then factor in the facts that we probably don't move as much in our fifties and sixties as we did in our teens and twenties, our protein intake might be down, and oxidative stress continues to build, and you can start to understand why menopause has a negative effect on muscle mass. Just to pile on, all of this adds up to gaining weight—by which I mean gaining fat. We also know that excess fat can increase the amount of oxidative stress, slowing us down even more—which in turn reduces our muscle-building capacity. I'm sure you're now getting the idea about the cycle of fat gain and muscle loss that menopause instigates.

As I hope you've gleaned by now, I'm usually pretty neutral about menopause's effects. They're natural and biological and nothing to feel bad about. But medically speaking, the loss of muscle is important because it has deleterious effects on one's quality of life. Even among younger people, muscle is a slow-growing tissue, and that growth grinds to a crawl in our older years for the reasons mentioned above. You're naturally inclined to move a little less than you did a couple decades ago. That's partly because of the loss of muscle mass—and it in turn *contributes* to the loss of muscle mass. Fat storage changes are altering your body in ways that you are forced to get used to, which can also have psychic effects on how much you want to get out and move your body.

Piling on here: Your muscle mass is a factor in your balance and co-ordination. If you have strong muscles (and healthy joints), you're able to compensate for tripping or a false move. Your body has fast-twitch muscles that are designed for moments like that. But if your muscles are degraded, you may not be able to regain your footing. And down you go. Your bones are not as durable as they once were—and you can see where I'm going with this. Older bodies aren't as bombproof as younger ones. They take longer to heal. And during that healing time, when a person's movements are limited, their muscle mass continues to degrade. You can see why a fall has such a cascading effect on an older person's life.

I'm sure you've seen this happen to people you love. I know I have. And it gives me a deeper level of compassion and appreciation for people who experience these sorts of injuries. But this is aging, which is a fact of life for all of us. It's not always pretty. It's not all doom and gloom, however. There are tons of healthy ways to cope so you can feel confident and capable as you weather this transition. But first, since I already alluded to joints, I want to quickly talk about those first.

The Effects on Joints

I'm not going to lie, joints are a common problem for people "of a certain age." We're talking about late forties, early fifties, and beyond. That's true of all people, menopausal or not. You go to the orthopedic surgeon for a joint replacement consultation, and the waiting room is filled with just as many men as women. Joints are the joining together of bones by connective tissue including cartilage, joint capsules, ligaments, and bursae. And these are slower-growing tissues, even in younger people.

However, the drags on muscle building that happen during menopause affect joints, too. Cartilage is a specialized building block of connective tissue, which is also a type of protein. And we know that our efficiency at turning protein into "body stuff"—muscle or connective tissue—declines because of the loss of estrogen. Not only that: estrogen is one of the body's great lubricators. So it makes sense that our joints are not going to be as well lubricated once our estrogen level drops.

Those are some of the gender-specific physiological differences that affect our joints. But then there's the reality that you've used these things for decades, and sometimes they degrade due to usage. And injuries don't necessarily heal on their own—something that is true for patients at every age.

A Note About Frozen Shoulder

I talk to my colleagues in the orthopedics community, and I've learned that shoulder synovitis—or frozen shoulder—is common among menopausal women. Studies back that up, as do my colleagues who treat the condition. It can be really devastating, especially when we are trying to move, stay fit, build muscle, improve our mood and sleep, and get blood flowing everywhere.

It's also something that happens to people who have had breast cancer. They may have a scar from a mastectomy or radiation therapy that left them with scar tissue. And scar tissue loves to proliferate, creating more scar tissue and basically having a party that reduces your mobility. I had my own journey with some of this, and to this day, I have had to work diligently to stretch the side of my radiated breast and scar. This is another reason why I am a huge fan of yoga, Pilates, and gyrotonics (therapeutic movement modality). Movement that focuses on weight bearing and flexibility in the context of more gentle stretching can be life changing—give it a try! Doing CrossFit may make you feel like a badass, but it will probably also hurt you.

The Fixes

Take Vitamin D Supplements

You'll remember from the previous section that vitamin D is a helper of bone growth. Muscle cells have receptors for vitamin D, too, so getting adequate amounts of it can help you maintain or increase your muscle mass. Remember when I talked about the fast-twitch muscle fibers that are important for stopping falls? People with adequate vitamin D levels have more fast-twitch, so-called Type II muscles. And in older people, maintaining adequate vitamin D levels improves physical performance, according to a study published in *Medicine & Science in Sports & Exercise* in 2009. Again, sunlight, certain cold-water fish, and fortified foods are among the things that can help increase your vitamin D levels, as can supplements.

Take DHEA Supplements

As I talked about earlier, DHEA is a prohormone—or precursor hormone—secreted by the adrenal gland. It is abundant earlier in life and declines as you age. It seems that it "indirectly exerts effects, among others, on bone formation, adiposity [fat storage], muscle, insulin and glucose metabolism, skin, libido, and well-being," according to a 2005 paper by researchers at the Laval University Hospital Research Center and Laval University in Québec, Canada. You and your doctor should determine together if you're a good candidate for DHEA supplementation. Again, it would be taken in conjunction with vitamin D.

Do Weight and Resistance Training

Usually I'm a proponent of exercise in any and all forms. But when it comes to muscle health, as with bone health, you get the most bang for your buck out of weight and resistance training. That means feeling the full weight of your body doing exercises such as squats and lunges and working out with resistance bands, dumbbells, kettlebells, and barbells—anything with some heft to it. (Contrast that with doing an activity such as aqua aerobics, which can increase your flexibility and get your heart rate up but does not support your body weight.)

The pressure on muscles as well as bones to perform under force is the distinguishing part of weight and resistance training. It's really key for tamping down on intramuscular fat and keeping your muscle tissue as healthy as possible (even if some amount of muscle mass decline is inevitable). A study published in 2009 in the journal *Menopause* took forty-eight postmenopausal women who fell into the BMI category of obese and put them into four groups. Some were led in resistance training for three months, some were put on a calorie-restrictive diet, some were doing resistance training and dieting, and finally there was the control group, just living their lives. After three months, the subjects who had done resistance training, as well as those who had done resistance training plus restricted their calorie intake, improved their overall body composition. Their body weight, total fat mass, percentage of fat mass, and body mass index were all reduced significantly. However, the people doing resistance training alone had the best improvement when it came to physical capacity. Having robust physical capacity is going to help the functioning of every system in your body, and having more muscle mass increases your metabolic rate.

Consider Your Protein Needs

Protein's main function in the body is as a builder. It's what makes up muscle, bones, and tissues. When you get injured, the body uses muscle to make repairs. There's been a lot of ink spilled in the last couple years on how much protein we need and whether Americans get enough of it. Like everything else having to do with nutrition, this is a highly individualized question, and, not to state the obvious, your protein intake will be influenced by the kind of diet you follow. In general, I would make sure that you're getting sufficient protein and spreading it out among your meals, rather than consuming it all at once; this will help your body utilize the protein you ingest more efficiently.

Let's spend a moment on the efficiency question. Because your body doesn't convert protein into muscle mass as efficiently after menopause, for a lot of people, it makes sense to try to compensate by increasing the amount of protein they're eating by a little bit. Whereas premenopausal people can get by with meeting the recommended daily allowance of 0.8 gram of protein for every kilogram of weight, research published in the *Journal of Nutrition, Health & Aging* in 2014 determined that postmenopausal woman should increase their intake to 1.1 grams of protein for every kilogram of weight.

Here's how you can find out how much that means for you:

First, convert your weight in pounds to kilograms. Since 2.2 pounds equals 1 kilogram, divide your weight by 2.2.

Second, multiply by 1.1. That equals the number of grams of protein you should aim for.

Here's the calculation for a 150-pound woman:

150 (weight in pounds)/2.2 (conversion to kilograms) = 68 kilograms
68 kilograms × 1.1 grams of protein = 74.8 grams of protein per day

---

Frequently Asked Question:
Should I Eat a High-Protein Diet?

I'm going to answer that question obliquely: *Be wary of extremes.* That goes for diet and exercise, and really anything else in your life with which you can go overboard. I'm seeing a lot of orthorexia, which is an unhealthy obsession with healthy eating. It's mentally unhealthy and can be linked to anxiety, depression, and even social isolation. And people who have orthorexia can actually get inadequate nutrition. It's one of those extremes that masks itself as a healthy lifestyle and is dangerous at any life stage.

To talk specifically about high protein, there's not great research out there involving postmenopausal women that says that high protein intake confers special health benefits. *Adequate* protein intake, yes, but not high protein intake.

Many, if not most, nutrition studies are done on men. High protein, high fat, intermittent fasting—those are just some of the diets with research that overlooks women. This likely goes back to something we've talked about: that researchers find it prohibitively complicated to take menstrual cycles into account, so they pack studies with nonmenstruating people. But we know that bodies that have the capacity for childbirth work differently. The hunger hormones leptin and ghrelin behave differently in men and women. So the truth is that not only do we lack sufficient evidence about postmenopausal diets, we don't have sufficient evidence for premenopausal diets! And I have one more bone to pick: a lot of the research out there about postmenopause centers around weight loss rather than eating for good health.

Now I'll address the keto elephant in the room: no, I do not support a keto diet. Again, there's no research saying that it's good for postmenopausal women. But hormonally, it doesn't make sense at this time in our lives. Once again, I am not into extremes. I think it's bad for eating, among other things. The good evidence, for both our own health and the health of the planet, says that we should be eating a plant-based diet.

By that I mean that 70 to 80 percent of what we eat should come from plants. We should also cut back on packaged foods as much as possible. Cardiac health is top of mind for me, and it should be for you, which means we really shouldn't be going whole hog (pun intended).

I know you want me to tell you exactly what to eat. But I'm a gynecologist and obstetrician, and my training in nutrition isn't extensive. I'm going to let you in on what is no longer a secret: doctors have almost zero nutrition training, and on the other hand, there are people who have amazing nutrition training. So if you're reading a book by an MD in a random field of medicine who tells you to, say, eat only red meat or stay away from oatmeal as though it's the plague, I would take it with a grain of salt. Instead, work with a nutritionist who holds the same values you do to assess what nutritional needs you have and figure out the best way to satisfy them. Individualized treatment and planning are always going to be the best course.

Here are a few things I can safely say. I like eating with Ayurveda in mind, which means eating seasonally, locally, and in as balanced a way as possible. For everyone, I recommend eating in a way that's sustainable for you, meaning you can continue doing so for the long haul, instead of following an intense, crazy diet that goes strong for a little while and then fizzles out hard. Eat with the planet in mind, too. And don't forget to have fun and enjoy! Personally, I don't find measuring and weighing all my food enjoyable—though if that works for you, cool, do it! But try not to weaponize food and what you consume. There's no such thing as good and bad foods. Stripping food of morality helps you eat a consistent diet that will work for you in the long run.

Limit or Nix Your Alcohol Intake

There's good evidence to suggest that heavier drinking may exacerbate sarcopenia. In a study that included 2,373 postmenopausal Korean women, published in the journal *Menopause* in 2017, sarcopenia was seen in 7.6 percent of the low-risk drinkers—riskiness relating to overall alcohol consumption—11 percent of the moderate-risk drinkers, and 22.7 percent of the high-risk drinkers. The high-risk drinkers were also more likely to smoke and had higher blood pressure and total cholesterol levels. If you're worried about your drinking or you think that your consumption could put you into the high-risk category, it might be time to scale back. There are resources that can help you do so. Hopefully you have a relationship with a doctor whom you trust and who can give you guidance. Talking to your loved ones about it, as well as a therapist, can help, too.

There are a few things you can do on your own to reduce or eliminate your drinking:

◆ Don't keep alcohol in the house.
◆ Write a list of the reasons you want to cut back, and read it when you feel yourself slipping.
◆ Have alcohol only one or two days a week—and don't binge on those days.
◆ Relocate group hangs from bars and beer gardens to museums or botanical gardens.
◆ Enter a twelve-step program to eliminate drinking and heal the wound that makes alcohol a tool of harm to your life and health. Go to meetings often enough to make sure your sobriety holds.

Heart Health and Heart Disease (Everybody Needs to Care About Their Ticker)

As a physician, I don't like to peddle fear. I also don't like to make sweeping generalizations, because each person's body is different. All of the things that make you *you*—they all started with different genetic predispositions. They were enhanced by a personal set of environmental factors and lifestyle decisions. If you happen to be blessed with an A+ genetic code for your cardiovascular system and every day for decades you've lived in a heart-smart way, then I suppose maybe you can skim through this next section. I've been into fitness since college, and when it comes to my own heart health, I'm still learning and adjusting my own habits. I hope you're open to doing so, too!

The caveat to all of these recommendations is that we actually don't know enough about the science of women's hearts! For generations, scientists just assumed that women's hearts were smaller versions of men's. That thinking persists even into today. I can't tell you how many women go in for heart imaging and the cardiologist will ask them, "Did you know you had a heart attack?" Women's hearts aren't the same as men's, and therefore the things that happen to women's hearts aren't the same. That helps explain why heart disease is the number one killer of women, accounting for about 20 percent of deaths. In fairness, it's also the number one killer of men; cardiac issues take the lives of 25 percent. Taken together, these statistics tell me that we all *think* we're taking better care of our hearts than we actually are. The good news is that once you start making cardiac care a priority, you'll start to experience positive changes almost immediately. We'll cover a lot of that in part IV.

Of course, I'm not a cardiologist, but I am a gynecologist. I look at heart issues through my unique lens. So I think the most useful thing I can offer is some overall advice that will, I hope, fundamentally change the way you think about cardiovascular health.

◆ **If you're between the ages of forty and fifty, you should see a primary care provider (PCP).** I can't tell you how many patients think that they can see me for everything. I can do a lot, but I'm not specifically looking at cardiac health—which is something your PCP will do. They're the ones looking at your history, evaluating tests, and ordering EKGs or chest X-rays. Preventive medicine is helpful for all the systems in the body, but it is *superimportant* for heart health. That is what your PCP is going to be able to provide.

◆ **Ninety-nine percent of you reading this book are not as heart healthy as you think.** Another thing that always comes up in my practice: people think that the heart issues that impacted their mother or grandmother aren't going to affect them. Here are some of the justifications I hear: "But she ate steak and potatoes every night!" "I go to spin class five times a week!" "She smoked for years!" These differences, yes, can help reduce your risk. But if you have a family history of cardiac issues, it's very hard to kale and sweat your way out. You really need to be followed by a doctor and follow their recommendations for surveillance or medications. One thing you can do proactively is know your family history. If your relatives are living, ask questions about their health background, including but not limited to heart issues.

◆ **Pregnancy is a stress test.** Have you heard this one? The basic idea is that carrying a baby puts a huge strain on your heart, so it's essentially a cardiac stress test. During pregnancy, your blood volume skyrockets to feed the growing uterus and placenta. This puts an enormous demand on the heart to pump more blood, as well as the blood vessels that act as channels for it—particularly the endothelium, which is the inner lining of those vessels. They are stretched to capacity. If you had a complications-free pregnancy, you passed the stress test. But if you had, say, preeclampsia, which is high blood pressure brought on by the pregnancy, or preterm delivery, I hate to sound harsh, but you failed the stress test. If that is the case, you need to be monitored by a cardiologist regularly, and they need to watch out for endothelial disease—a form of coronary artery disease—among other things.

The same goes for gestational diabetes. If you had gestational diabetes, you have a 50 percent risk of developing type 2 diabetes later in life. You need to be more careful about preventing insulin resistance by avoiding excess sugar and carbs, and you have to stick to an exercise plan—because we know that insulin resistance is also bad for the heart.

◆ **Trouble getting pregnant could be a warning sign, too.** If you suffered from fertility issues or recurrent pregnancy losses, that can be an indicator of an autoimmune disease or an inflammatory issue, both of which can be a drag on your heart. Your gynecologist, PCP, and cardiologist can look for ways to bolster your heart health to avoid cardiac disease down the line.

Gynecologic and Breast Cancers (Information Is Empowering)

Here's what I'm not going to do: I'm not going to lecture you about all of the different gynecological cancers. If you, like me, end up being diagnosed with one, you will become an expert in your particular brand of cancer, whether you want to or not. What I think would be much more helpful is a practical list of things you can do to decrease your risk of cancer or aid in its early detection. Sound good? Here's how.

◆ **Look at your vulva.** Yes, this is the hand mirror situation. Getting to know what your exterior genitalia look like will make you equipped to notice changes, such as color changes, bumps or raised areas, and texture differences. Do this about once a month. And just know that, as you age, things *will* change!

◆ **Get the human papillomavirus (HPV) vaccine.** Human papillomavirus is a sexually transmitted infection that can lead to cancer, and there is a vaccine for it. It's now approved for people up to age forty-six. It's safe and effective. There's no reason not to get it.

◆ **Be honest with your provider about the kind of sex you're having.** This is related to HPV. If you're having anal sex, your gynecologist should be checking your perineum and anus for signs of HPV—something that is both common and often overlooked.

◆ **If you are having abnormal bleeding, go to your gynecologist now.** If you are still menstruating, this means you are bleeding through a tampon, pad, or cup in less than thirty to sixty minutes. If your periods are getting closer together—meaning that you're menstruating every three weeks—it's a good time to make an appointment. If you are postmenopausal and begin bleeding, you should also make an appointment. These could be signs of uterine (endometrial) cancer, which is very treatable when caught early. I should mention that they are also classic symptoms of fibroids, adenomyosis or endometriosis, and endometrial polyps, all of which are noncancerous.

◆ **If you are having watery discharge, go to your gynecologist now.** Watery discharge that seems to come out of the blue could be a sign of fallopian tube cancer or possibly ovarian cancer. If you're noticing this, don't skip ahead to the worst possible outcome. But take the reins of your health and get it checked out.

Frequently Asked Question: Should I Get Genetic Testing?

This is a question I answer often, and it's always asked with trepidation, because a genetic test will reveal one of two things: either you have a genetic predisposition for a certain disease or diseases, or you don't. My answer is typically: if you're going to do something about it, then yes. Meaning, if the result comes in that you *do* have a genetic predisposition and you are prepared to make proactive decisions about screening and potentially preventive surgery to reduce or eliminate that risk, you are a better candidate for genetic testing. However, getting results and not acting on them just invites worry into your life.

That said, there are a few instances when genetic testing is recommended. For instance, if you were diagnosed with colon cancer at an unusually young age, you may want to get genetic testing to see if it's related to a genetic defect that also sets you up for other cancers. That way you will have access to the screening you need.

Even if you have a strong family history of a certain disease, the results of a test are not a given. For example, a family history of breast cancer does not necessarily mean that you have a BRCA mutation. It doesn't mean that you *don't* have a genetic predisposition for breast cancer, either. You could have a mutation on a part of the genome whose breast cancer link has not yet been identified, or the mutation could be unique to your family.

All of that brings me to my last point: if you're going to do genetic testing, *you must absolutely 100 percent of the time participate in genetic counseling as well.* Even doctors who get genetic testing do this. The counselor is trained in using the results of the genetic test, as well as information you as the patient provide about your family tree, to give you a full picture of your genetic predispositions to certain diseases and recommend where you should go from there.

Breast Cancer: Healthy Living, Healthy Vigilance

As you no doubt know, around one in eight women gets breast cancer, and yours truly is one of them. If you become a member of this club, we're so sorry you're here, but we're going to take good care of you.

Estrogen plays a role in a lot of breast cancers, but not all. Family history and genetic factors play a role in a lot of breast cancers, but not all. Therefore I'm not going to describe every possible scenario with its corresponding outcome and treatment. It would be overwhelming and not really necessary. If you've ever had cancer or another big medical event, you know that you become an expert in your own disease anyway, so I'd just like to make a few recommendations.

Get Your First Mammogram by Age Forty

Guidelines have been changing as to the age when you should get your first mammogram. In the past couple years, some of the professional groups that create these sorts of guidelines adjusted the age of a person's first mammogram downward. You might say, well that's a good idea! Make it younger, find more cancer, right? The problem is that when younger people get mammograms, they may inadvertently uncover more false positives or even very small tumors that the body would clear by itself. We don't like false positives because they create unnecessary psychological burdens, and we worry about catching cancers when they're too small (believe it or not) because of the fear of overtreatment. As we get older, the chance that masses are something to worry about goes up, and the ability for the body to clear malignancies by itself drops. The advantages are that, yes, earlier mammograms will inevitably catch some cancers earlier. Your first mammogram creates a baseline for breast imaging moving forward. All of us docs pretty much agree that you should be getting annual mammograms starting at age forty.

This is, of course, for women who have a normal risk of developing breast cancer. If you're in a high-risk group because of a genetic predisposition, your family history, or having had other cancers, your doctor may recommend that you start mammograms or other breast imaging screening earlier.

Perform Monthly Breast Self-Exams

Breast self-exams are truly an act of self-care. No one knows your body better than you do, so you're the best equipped to notice changes. I'm going to crib from the National Breast Cancer Foundation and share that organization's three simple steps for a breast self-exam:

1. **In the shower.** With the pads/flats of the three middle fingers on your left hand and your right arm behind your head, check the entire right breast and armpit area, pressing down with light, medium, and firm pressure. Repeat on the opposite side, with your right hand on your left breast, feeling for lumps, thickening, hardened knots, and any other breast changes.

2. **In front of a mirror.** First, visually inspect your breasts with your arms at your sides. Next, raise your arms high overhead. Look for any changes in the contour, any swelling or dimpling of the skin, and any changes in the nipples. Next, rest your palms on your hips and press firmly to flex your chest muscles. Your left and right breasts will not exactly match—few women's do—so look for any dimpling, puckering, or changes, particularly on one side.

3. **Lying down.** When you lie down, your breast tissue spreads out evenly along the chest wall. Place a pillow under your right shoulder and your right arm behind your head. Using your left hand, move the pads of your fingers around your right breast over the entire breast area and armpit. Use light, medium, and firm pressure. Squeeze the nipple, checking for discharge and lumps. Repeat these steps for your left breast.

Eat Healthfully and Exercise

The same diet guidelines that are good for your bones, hot flashes, and skin are also good for your breasts. Drink as little alcohol as possible, and, as with smoking cigarettes, if you can cut drinking out entirely, all the better. Eat fresh fruits and vegetables; a colorful diet means you're getting a variety of vitamins and antioxidants. Move your body every day. Weight lifting, cardio, and stretching/recovery will keep your body in tip-top shape.

Of course, we all know people who did everything right: never smoked, had a glass of Champagne on special occasions only, ran 10Ks, meditated—and still got cancer. It happens All. The. Time. The reaction isn't, however, to throw up your hands, say "Screw it," and go to town on a bag of Funyuns. If you do all of those things and then get cancer, your body is at a better baseline to withstand the physical demands of surgery and treatment, as well as the emotional toll that comes with a cancer diagnosis.

Alzheimer's Disease and Dementia
(They're Scary, Yes. But There Are
Things We Can Do About Them)

It might surprise you to know that nearly two-thirds of Alzheimer's patients are women. It's a fact not much talked about, and that blind spot is reflected in the research. So many studies—too many—in the past few decades have been agnostic to gender, meaning that researchers haven't been studying the biological underpinnings that make Alzheimer's more prevalent among women. In fact, the organization Women's Health Access Matters (WHAM), along with the RAND Corporation, released a report in April 2021 that found that in 2019, only 12 percent of the National Institutes of Health's Alzheimer's disease research budget was devoted to projects that focused specifically on women.

It seems that Alzheimer's may be underdiagnosed among women, too. A paper published in the journal *Neurology* in 2016 found that women seem to possess a "sex-specific cognitive reserve" and that verbal memory decline related to neural dysfunction doesn't show up until the disease has advanced.

If you know someone who's battled Alzheimer's or it runs in your family, the possibility of developing it can be a really scary prospect, especially since research hasn't resulted in any viable, reliable treatment options. But there are advancements being made in understanding why menopause seems to act as a trigger for Alzheimer's. For instance, Lisa Mosconi, PhD, the director of the Women's Brain Initiative, associate director of the Alzheimer's Prevention Clinic at Weill Cornell Medical College/New York-Presbyterian Hospital, and author of *The XX Brain: The Groundbreaking Science Empowering Women to Maximize Cognitive Health and Prevent Alzheimer's Disease*, has studied positron emission tomography (PET) scans of women's brains to see how the menopausal transition changes brain metabolism. The brain's preferred source of energy is glucose, or sugar. Researchers including Dr. Mosconi track brain function via the metabolism rate. As a person gets further along in their menopause transition, their brain glucose metabolism begins to slow. As we know, estrogen is great at doing a lot of things, including regulating brain metabolism. The working theory is that the change in brain bioenergetics has to do with the sudden drop in estrogen.

What happens when brain glucose metabolism slows down? Though the brain prefers to use glucose for energy, it can metabolize lipids instead—though that's our gray matter's last resort. "Lipids constitute the bulk of the dry mass of the brain and have been associated with healthy function as well as the most common pathological conditions of the brain," write researchers in *Frontiers in Physiology*. So energy metabolism in the brain seems to be an important piece of the puzzle. Other research is looking into tau proteins, which are tangled proteins inside cells that inhibit their proper function. *APOE4* is a gene variant that seems to increase the risk of Alzheimer's, and women with that variant tend to develop Alzheimer's faster than do men who have the variant.

There's a lot of ground to cover when it comes to Alzheimer's, in terms of both the disease itself and the treatment opportunities. Across the country, researchers are looking into things such as immune system function related to cognitive decline, gut microbiome–brain connections, and further decoding genes to predict future Alzheimer's disease.

However, that does not mean we're helpless in reducing our risk of getting Alzheimer's. In 2020, a report by The Lancet Commission was released that updated the risk factors for dementia and categorized them by the age group when the risk factors come into play. The commission estimated that these twelve modifiable risks account for around 40 percent of worldwide dementias. Here's what it found:

Early life (under age 45)

◆ Less education

Midlife (ages 45 to 65)

◆ Hearing loss
◆ Traumatic brain injury
◆ Hypertension
◆ Consumption of more than twenty-one units of alcohol per week
◆ Obesity, with a body mass index greater than 30

Later life (over age 65)

◆ Smoking
◆ Depression
◆ Social isolation
◆ Physical inactivity
◆ Diabetes
◆ Air pollution

Rather than talking about each risk factor individually, I want to make some overall recommendations.

Take Part in Activities That You Enjoy and That Challenge Your Mind

The panel referenced research revealing that "travel, social outings, playing music, art, physical activity, reading, and speaking a second language, were associated with maintaining cognition, independent of education, occupation, late-life activities, and current structural brain health." What does this tell me? Well, childhood education is well behind you, as are other possibilities for cognitive development that are age dependent. However, there are ways to keep your brain healthy, no matter your age. The big takeaway is that it's never too late. Sign up for a language class at the community college. Join a book club. Take an art class. Anything that invigorates your mind is great. You get bonus points if you do it with others. Connection with people helps combat feelings of loneliness or isolation, which we know are detrimental to both emotional and physical health.

Eat a Mostly Plant-Based Diet, and Get Moving

Diabetes and high blood pressure are risk factors for Alzheimer's and dementia, as they are for other diseases. Curb your refined sugar intake as much as possible (natural sources of sugar, such as berries, are fine), and eat a plant-based diet as often as you can. Alcohol consumption should be limited or nixed. I'm not going to berate you again about smoking—you know what to do. And exercise, which is important for blood flow to all parts of your body, including your brain.

Get Your Hearing Checked, and Use Hearing Aids if You Need Them

Hearing loss and dementia seem to be closely linked, possibly due to reduced cognitive stimulation. The worse hearing loss gets, the higher the risk of developing dementia. If you don't think your hearing is what it used to be, tell your doctor, who may refer you to a hearing loss specialist. If it turns out that you need hearing aids, I'd recommend you get them. There's still a lot of self-consciousness about hearing loss, but I hope you'll agree that the payoff of being able to hear outweighs the social discomfort. Plus, hearing aids are getting smaller and more discreet. Taking care of your hearing is more than just staving off dementia; it's about staying connected and engaged.

Frequently Asked Question:
Is Brain Fog the Same as Dementia?

No. This is a question that comes up because brain fog commonly crops up during the menopausal transition. Hormone changes occurring during menopause, thyroid issues, stress, fatigue, and depression can all contribute to brain fog. I know from firsthand experience that it's incredibly frustrating and sometimes embarrassing. But brain fog often clears up. However, if you're having memory issues and having trouble functioning in your day-to-day life in ways that used to come easily—such as taking care of your finances, doing household chores, and taking part in social activities—these may suggest cognitive decline. Talk to your doctor about what you're experiencing. Those things, coupled with risk factors such as a history of traumatic brain injuries or the prevalence of Alzheimer's in your family, may warrant looking into a further investigation of your cognitive status.

Symptoms Worksheet

When you visit your doctor with this worksheet in hand, they will be over the moon. We have a much easier time giving you care if we have the data we need.

Hot Flashes

- How often are you hot flashing? How many days a week or times a day?
- On a scale of 1 to 10, how bad are the hot flashes? Are you able to feel yourself getting warm but it doesn't change what you're doing (1), or do you need to remove yourself from what you're doing and give yourself an opportunity to recover (10)?

Sleep Disruption

- How often do you wake up in the middle of the night?
- Do you know why you are waking up? Is it due to night sweats? Is it due to a need to urinate? Is it due to something else?
- Do you have problems falling asleep? On average, how long does it take you to fall asleep?
- Do you have problems staying asleep? How long does it take you to fall back asleep once you've woken up?

Genitourinary Syndrome of Menopause (GSM)

- Do you have vulvar discomfort while you're doing everyday activities, such as walking or biking?

- Is penetrative sex or masturbation uncomfortable or painful? Are you experiencing bleeding afterward?
- If you've tried a lubricant for either everyday use or use during sex, does it work for you? What has your experience been like?
- How has urination changed for you? Does the need to urinate go straight to a bathroom emergency? Is urination uncomfortable? Do you leak during activities such as coughing, laughing, running, or jumping?
- Have you noticed any physical or visual changes to your genitals?

Weight Gain

- How are you feeling in your body? Has that been changing during your menopausal transition?
- What kind of exercise do you do? How often? When you exercise consistently, how does it make you feel?

Hair, Skin, Teeth, and Nails

- Have you noticed that your hair texture or durability is changing? What about your nails?
- Do you have a dermatologist you like? Do you see them for skin checks?
- What about going to the dentist? Are you getting cleanings and checkups?

Bone, Muscle, and Joint Health

- Are you noticing any pain or discomfort during movement?
- If you do get injured, what do you do to ease the pain? How long does it take to heal?

Overall

◆ How are you feeling emotionally? Are you experiencing depressive symptoms, such as a lack of motivation, sadness, or fatigue? If so, how many days a week? How is it impacting your day-to-day life? For instance, does it stop you from going out with friends and family?

◆ What is your favorite physical activity? How often do you do it? Do you move every day or almost every day?

◆ Does what you're eating make you feel good? Does it help you have sustained energy throughout the day, or does your energy level spike and dip?

◆ Are there changes happening in your body—any changes—that you're curious about or that are causing you worry? Menopause can be at the root of lots of these. Sometimes there's a fix, sometimes not. But bring them up with your doctor regardless!

PART III

But How Are You *Really* Doing?

*The "feelings" side of menopause can make you
feel alone. I'm here to tell you that you're not.*

Because I can't help but take my work home with me, I was thinking of the menopausal transition while sitting in a darkened theater watching the movie *Wonder Woman*. It's heralded as a comic book feminist anthem. I'm not on board. This feeling started during the opening scene of the movie, when the camera pans over Themyscira, the island nation of Diana, soon to be Wonder Woman. Little girls are running around freely, and young women are in training to be warriors under the tutelage of those a generation or so older. There is not a lot of body diversity. Of course, there's not a man in sight. I went home afterward and learned more about Themyscira. This seemed like an occasion to trust Wikipedia.

"Themyscira is a segregated nation of women—regarded as a feminist utopia—governed by *Aphrodite's Law*, which declared that the Amazons would be immortal as long as no man sets foot on their island," the Wiki writers tell me. "Men are banned from Themyscira under penalty of death. Themyscira's location is undisclosed; as a security measure, the island can shift its location over both land and time, remains undetectable from the perspective of any outside observer, and as soon as anyone leaves the island, they forget its location."

There's . . . a lot to unpack here. And I realize that some of the trappings of this Paradise Island were created back in the 1940s and the idea was for it to be a foil to the aggressive, male-dominated workplaces where women were often uninvited—or, at best, in which they were background actors. Themyscira was both ahead of its time in its desire to create a feminist utopia, as well as a little bit of a blunt object (I'm not thinking that its creator, William Moulton Marston, aka Charles Moulton, was considering trans people or those who are gender fluid or nonbinary or the fact that contact with men does not irrevocably taint women). But I kept asking myself, where are the older gals? The leaders in Themyscira were not wizened, gray-haired ladies. They were, in Earth years, maybe in their forties or early fifties. They all had the physiques of American Ninja Warriors. It's hard not to be in awe of them. But still, there was something missing.

I was thinking about all this on the way home. It was an *aha!* moment. Were there really no old ladies in the film? I searched my memory for people with deep groove lines across their faces denoting age and experience, handicapped seating in the amphitheater for those who couldn't leap to their feet, anyone with snow-white hair. But what had I been expecting, anyway? It's a fantasy world within a comic book movie that's marketing itself widely to get big returns at the box office (which means that as feminist as it wants to be, the actors are going to have to show some skin), so maybe I shouldn't be so hypercritical. On the other hand, it says something that Themyscira would be entirely without old ladies. Implied in that is that if you're going to live forever, you want to do so in Gal Gadot's body. Because I'm thinking that Gal Gadot gets out of bed without her knees creaking. (And Gal, if you read this, I'm not trying to objectify you, but I am almost certain that the stunt training you endured did not involve "make ankle circles and pedal legs before getting out of bed.")

So there they are, the inhabitants of Themyscira, living in a form of perpetual youth. And here I am, thinking how great it would be to go through menopause there, surrounded by people who understand you and won't judge you if your face suddenly flushes and you stick a bag of frozen peas on the back of your neck. If Themyscira had people going through the menopausal transition, I bet the city would even have cooling areas scented with lavender or eucalyptus. Lubricants and supplements would be made free for all who need them. And if we're going to create a later-in-life fantasy world, memories would stay intact and no one would need an oncologist. They would still be viewed as sexual and vivacious. Those who are in the menopausal transition would be revered for the wisdom they've amassed and the lessons they embody.

*   *   *

If we were all together at an in-person bootcamp, at this point I'd ask if people wanted to share any thoughts from their own lives. To get things started, I want to share mine. I'm actually writing this in the car, on a cross-country road trip with my daughter, the younger of my two children. The back seat of the car is crammed with all of her things to move back into college in New York State after a pandemic year spent at home in Los Angeles. No one had had an easy time. She hadn't, I hadn't, nor had her brother or my partner. The four of us had lived together intensely, as everyone did during that time—for better and worse. I had been the only one leaving the house to go to work, which was both liberating and perilous.

She's moving into an apartment. I am excited to be here, but my anxiety is making an appearance. It's something that I started to notice a few years ago. I have always been adept at juggling. You don't have kids during residency and raise them with an out-of-work, soon-to-be ex-husband while seeing patients, delivering babies day and night, and trying to practice some modicum of self-care to stave off burnout without learning how to juggle. And I'm juggling now. Trying to finish this book. Working on getting a new health start-up off the ground. Working with my partners at the practice to transition out of the obstetrics practice. (I love obstetrics, and I would attend births for the rest of my life, but the unpredictable schedule and stretches of sleepless nights are taking a toll on my body and I can't cope with it anymore, physically or mentally.)

My mom died last year. It was during the pandemic, but it wasn't related to the pandemic.

And I'm certainly in the menopausal transition. That I know, although I wasn't the first to notice it. It was my medical assistant who did. I was in my early forties, and all told she had worked for me for seven years. In that time we became close. One day I woke up and realized that I had been snippy and snappy to everyone around me, including at work. Things that at one time hadn't gotten to me really raised my ire. People bugged me. It was understandable, as I had little kids at home and a husband who was out of work. (Honestly, the marriage was not good, either.) But shit really got to me at the same time every month. It was, you guessed it, PMS.

"I'm so sorry!" I told my medical assistant. "I didn't realize it until now."

"That's okay. I knew you were just getting your period," she generously replied.

I had never dealt with PMS, nor with the insane cramps that were now trying to kill me with every menstrual cycle. I finally made the connection between those and the breast tenderness I'd been having that was so strong that I could've sworn I was pregnant. For years, I would never admit to my patients that I was one of those lucky people for whom periods were never a big deal. They came, I bled, they went. No cramps, no mood disruptions. Now my body was changing. I did some research and started to take an herbal supplement called chasteberry, which has been used for breast tenderness, PMS, and polycystic ovarian syndrome, among other things. It worked well for me, and I recommended it to some patients, many of whom had success taking it. That experience accelerated some thinking I'd done for decades, since my first foray into complementary medicine. All through my years of being a doctor and developing a specialty in taking care of people going through menopause, I had wondered what my own transition would be like. Would I opt for menopausal hormone treatment, or would I be drawn to my Ayurvedic training and rely on herbs? I'm generally an open-minded person, and I treat myself like I treat my patients; I respond to what's happening now while keeping future health in mind. I find an appropriate response and am flexible enough to try things for a while, decide what is and isn't working, and move on when necessary. That approach had worked throughout my life, so why shouldn't it now? When it came to my own menopausal transition, I was quietly confident. Who better to ride into this next phase of life than the person who partners with so many patients going through it?

And then I got cancer. And got divorced.

I've talked about my breast cancer already, but I want to put it into the context of my menopause journey. Cancer changed my body. The biggest outer change is the big radiation scar on my breast. I'll be honest, there are days that it's hard to look at. And the scar tissue underneath has made movement at times very uncomfortable or restricted. Up until recently I was taking a drug called tamoxifen, an estrogen-blocking drug that's prescribed to reduce the chances of a breast cancer recurrence. Some people do really well on tamoxifen. I was not one of them. Over the course of the eighteen months that I took tamoxifen, the drug made me feel horrible and accelerated or magnified some of the menopause symptoms, such as mood changes, joint pain, and vaginal dryness. I did what doctors do and dived into the research. Then, with the blessing of my oncologist, I decided to take a yearlong holiday because my joint pain was so severe that I could no longer lift heavy weights or exercise in a meaningful way, and *that* was the key to both my mental health and recovery.

I restarted and completed five years on tamoxifen and then discontinued it due to newer research and genotype testing indicating that five more years of the suppression that the drug provides would not significantly improve my prognosis. I individualized my treatment with the guidance of my doctor, evolving evidence, and an eye on my own personal, day-to-day experience. To be clear, *I am not recommending suspending tamoxifen for you.* Nor am I saying that you should stay on it forever and I got a hall pass. The wisdom of the story is in how the decisions were made over the course of many years. My thinking and my medical team's process evolved with my medical and lifestyle needs and followed research advancements. I had the opportunity to make these nuanced treatment decisions because of an oncology partner who was open to having conversations. And yes, the fact that I'm a doctor made it easier to have them. But if you aren't a doctor, that should not stop you from having the same kind of care partnership. I know, because that is the relationship I have with my patients. It's that kind of processing and decision making that I wish for everyone.

With my breast cancer under control and my feet more firmly planted beneath me than they'd been in years, I decided to date again—as a divorced parent of two, while still working as a partner at a big practice and continuing the process of healing. And going through the menopausal transition. Even with all of that going on, making human connections was important to me as someone who thrives on them—though I was feeling a little shaky over the prospect of dating again. Feeling a little unsure of myself, I consulted a close friend couple. Gingerly, I confided that I was worried that the breast cancer scar would be a turnoff. The wife had some soothing words for me about what I'd been through and how I would be seen as a resilient and empathetic partner.

Then her husband piped up, "If you take your clothes off, the only thing in a man's brain is 'BOOBS! BOOBS! BOOBS!'" I did indeed find a partner. And the scar has never been a turnoff.

*   *   *

I am absolutely not asking for your sympathy in all of this. There are many people who are struggling out there, and I recognize that I have immense amounts of privilege that make whatever my struggles are easier by virtue of my outward appearance, my sexual and gender identity, my family history, and the economic stability that comes from generational wealth. I'm telling you this because there may be parts of my story that feel connected to yours, regardless of your status of privilege. There aren't a lot of universals, but two of them are that everyone with a vulva has, by the time they get to menopause, experienced some sort of trauma related to medicine; and everyone has a story to tell, and it feels better to share it versus keeping it bottled up inside.

I practice what I preach. The Menopause Bootcamp, like my medical practice, relies on honesty and acknowledging the mind-body-spirit connections. It is a space where we can be candid about the times the medical establishment has failed us. Given how much you know about my body, you might be surprised to learn that I am a fairly private person. What has evolved in my own mind is that some of those things that I felt were so private and intimate just don't feel that way anymore. Every day I hear from patients who are having feelings and experiences that make them feel isolated. And the isolation—and the shame—act to multiply their symptoms. Physical symptoms can turn into psychological ones and vice versa. Sometimes patients come in with a complaint that they'd been keeping bottled up. Maybe it's a new anxiety that they've developed, a skin change that bothers them, a reduction in libido that takes them by surprise. Then they're caught off guard when I say, "Yes, that makes sense! I see you, and I hear you. You're not alone in this." We go through a list of the options available to address this new thing, and you'd be surprised how often they don't really do anything about it. After all of that worry, they essentially let it ride. It's not because they are unmotivated to put the solutions into motion or that the cost of the solutions is too high; it's because what they really wanted was to be seen and heard and their experience validated. Medicine isn't always this way. Everyone walks down a long road, and it doesn't always end in health and tranquility. But being connected is grounding. Feeling validated is reassuring. I know that from my own experience. By reading this book, you have become the newest member of the Menopause Bootcamp. It's now up to you to make those around you feel connected and validated and ask the same of them when you need it.

Lessons from the Chrysalis

While writing this book, I interviewed people who have different lived experiences to better understand more perspectives. The metaphor of the menopausal transition's being like a chrysalis came up *a lot*. As you probably remember from elementary school, caterpillars go through a pupa stage before becoming butterflies. The little sac that they're in, the chrysalis, is weirder than we were led to believe when we were ten years old. After the caterpillar entombs itself in its shell, its body breaks down into a goo. It's a gnarly transformation. And yes, in a week or two, it emerges as a butterfly, but even that is a birthlike process and a painstaking one. Watch a YouTube video of the process, and you really feel for the butterfly. Nature is not known to be gentle. But at the end, the new creature that emerges has *wings*! It sees the world from a different perspective—from on high! Butterflies are pollinators, so they drink up the nutritious nectar from wildflowers and bushes; in doing so, they leave behind pollen that their feet have picked up from other plants and thus help plants reproduce, making the world better for other butterflies and insects. It's fucking beautiful when you think of it like that.

I imagine that if caterpillars had bigger brains, they wouldn't look forward to the chrysalis phase—especially those that were claustrophobic. But their butterfly elders would remind them that transformation is difficult—both physically and spiritually—but is an essential part of their lives. Plus, I like to think that knowing that you'd end up developing wings and seeing the world from an incredible new perspective would make it a celebrated experience.

Menopause is a transformation. So much of what we've been talking about so far and how you might be feeling—that's the good part of it. Then there are the uncomfortable, sometimes painful parts. I'm reminded of an anecdote that one of the leaders of the American Ayurveda community and a founder of the National Ayurvedic Medical Association, Light Miller, shared at a conference. During her own menopause transition, she made a ritual for herself: she crafted a cave in her home and stayed there alone for an extended amount of time to pray, fast, and meditate. She created a difficult and intense ritual to mark the time and emerged from her cramped, dark cave with a different perspective. It's extreme but fascinating.

What I have realized, both in my own experience and in talking with people who have gone through it, is that the discomfort isn't gratuitous; it has a purpose. A lot of us realize that the patterns we developed in the previous three or four decades of life aren't working anymore. People who were raised as cis girls were inculcated from a young age to be caregivers—to give of themselves and not necessarily ask for the same in return. The menopausal transition can be an opportunity to reflect on that pattern and decide if it's fulfilling for you. For some, it is! I'm not trying to judge. But the menopause years are an opportunity for self-assessment.

I'm going to get real with you: I've struggled with the body changes that I've noticed, and they have forced me to rethink some of the hang-ups I have harbored for probably my whole life. I transformed from a pudgy kid into an athletic young adult and have cultivated a body to match for thirty years. Now I'm getting heavier, and the skin on my décolletage is crepier than it's ever been. That shouldn't bother me. I know our conceptions around our own bodies are shaped by societal standards of youth and beauty as seen through the lens of the patriarchy. But it doesn't stop me from wondering if I'm still alluring to my man. I'm not the only one who harbors such feelings. Maybe for you it manifests itself in a never-ending desire to lose ten more pounds. Or the belief that if you just had the right green juice concoction your skin would be bright and firm. That you'll finally get onto a dating site once you work on your arms/abs/thighs a little more. Menopause forces us to let that shit go. Doing so can hurt. Change hurts. Change that's forced upon us hurts worse. It breaks us down, turns us into goo—and sets us up for the transformation.

As for myself, I'm getting there. My self-consciousness is waning, replaced by feelings of pride, peace, and self-forgiveness. It's a journey, for sure. There are days that are great, some that are slogs, and many more that lie somewhere between the two.

I know your head is probably swimming with all of the information you read in the last part. There's a physical reality to menopausal changes that is overwhelming. And I'd like to talk about that feeling and anything else you're feeling about this transition.

But we've got to get to the bottom of where all of these feelings are coming from if we are to address them properly. What I mean is that not all of them will have fixes. We've already discussed that it is disorienting to realize that the body you've been accustomed to for decades is changing and you are trying to figure out who you are now. There's no fix for that. It doesn't mean that we shouldn't talk about it; we have to. But no supplement or prescription drug can take the place of spending time discovering your new body.

CHAPTER 4

The Mind-Body Connection

Have you heard the term *gynechiatrist*? Like a hairdresser, a gynecologist ends up acting as a kind of psychiatrist stand-in because she learns a lot about her patients, and not just the medical stuff. Patients are apt to speak candidly about how they're feeling, and it's an honor to be a trusted person for my patients. In fact, ob-gyns can play an important role in detecting, preventing, and treating depression, since we see our patients during vulnerable times in their lives, including adolescence, pregnancy, postpartum, and the menopausal transition, according to 2017 research from the University of Washington in Seattle.

Mental health isn't my specialty, however, so although there is a lot I can do, there are some patients to whom I recommend seeing a therapist and possibly a psychiatrist, who is a medical doctor and can prescribe medication. It goes without saying that if my patients are showing signs of a mental health crisis—such as thinking about harming themselves or others—there is an emergency protocol to get those people the help they need. If this rings true for you or someone you know, please talk to a physician immediately or call the National Suicide Prevention Lifeline at 800-273-8255.

Even if you're not at the point where major intervention is required, menopause is almost always a time when mental health issues crop up. I'll take myself as an example. When I was going through the menopausal transition, I had some crazy bouts of PMS symptoms. My short fuse led to fights at home. I might have picked a fight with my colleagues. There was some car crying. Some car eating. My body was tired from the long hours at work as well as the changes happening, and my mind was really tired, too. Luckily, I had the tools to understand what was going on and what might have been exacerbating the way I was feeling. That's what I want to share with you now: a checklist with solutions that will work for just about everyone. What we know about mental health issues and depressive symptoms—anxiety, loss of interest or pleasure, mood swings, hopelessness, agitation, social isolation, irritability, and fatigue, among others—is that they are typically multifactorial. No one thing is causing you to feel this way. My approach, then, is to address some of the universal habits or conditions that may be causing you to feel the way you do. Once those are on their way to being resolved, you can discover what is happening that's unique to you and your life that's causing you distress.

After that, we'll explore some of the specific feelings of people who go through menopause. Some of them will feel germane to you, others won't. But when we learn about other people's experiences, it gives us more empathy.

The whole process brings to mind the beautiful wood beams in the vaulted ceiling of my classic 1920s Spanish Revival living room. When we renovated the home, which had housed three families in the past hundred years, we removed twenty-six layers of paint and stain and got a history lesson along the way. The first thing you do is take a big sander and get off as much of the caked-on paint as you can. Each layer that comes off gets you closer to revealing what lives underneath. And it's a process. After the big sander comes finer-gauge sanders, then specialized tools that can gently remove more of the wood's covering, until you finally learn what the foundation looks like, what it's made of. That's the way I approach mental health for my patients and for myself. There are big, universal things that we should all be doing that can help reduce depression. These don't get to the root cause, however; that comes later.

Since you may not be into home restoration, let's just dive right into the hierarchy.

CHAPTER 5

Physical Foundations of Mental Health

I want to ask you a series of questions that I go through with almost all my patients periodically. Then I'll provide some insights into why your answers illuminate how you're feeling.

How's Your Sleep?

Are you getting between seven and nine hours of sleep a night? Are you able to fall asleep easily? Stay asleep? Do you feel well rested when you awaken, and can you function well throughout the day?

Why it's so important: Nothing—*nothing*—good is going to happen in your life if you don't get enough sleep. Yes, you can tell me about supersleepers who subsist on a few hours a night. There are very few of them, though, so chances are that you are not one of them. The effective amount and pattern of sleep for you is based on your chronotype, meaning the way your individual circadian rhythm operates. Some people feel great after six hours of sleep; others need eight; a handful of you may do well with four-hour chunks. But you need enough of whatever is right for you. Everyone has a threshold, and if you go below that, you feel crappy.

Listen, I know what it's like to try to function in this world on too little shut-eye. It's called being a doctor. Our training has us in a constant state of inadequate sleep. And you can talk to my partner or my kids: you do not want to be around me after I've been on an overnight shift at the hospital. I have zero patience. I don't feel well. I'm not firing on all cylinders. My emotions can swing easily. It's *brutal*. You've already read about how important sleep is, and in part II you learned some of the things you can do to improve sleep. But I want to say plainly that if you are feeling mentally unwell, you need to prioritize sleep.

I recognize that for some people, mood symptoms such as anxiety and depression are part of the reasons they *can't* sleep. Which is a sticky wicket; the fix for sleep is the reason you can't sleep. In that case, we need to get to the root of some of that anxiety and depression. Is it related to night sweats, which is something we can address? Do you have a medical condition or conditions that need attention, such as sleep apnea or cardiovascular disease, that are causing you to sleep poorly? Are you having gastrointestinal problems, such as constipation or GI distress after eating meals or drinking? These can be directly related to anxiety and depression, and we need to think about them!

I was speaking to a mentor of mine named Mary Thompson, an incredible Ayurvedic practitioner. She told me about a woman she was working with who was complaining of poor sleep, constipation, and headaches. Ayurveda teaches us that everything that goes on in the body has links to the gut and the mind and that we need to address those first. So Mary wanted to relieve this woman's constipation.

"But I'm more concerned about the sleep and the headaches," the client told Mary.

"Just give me one week," Mary replied. Before the seven days were up, the client's constipation was resolved, and so were the sleep disturbances and headaches.

Now, a doctor trained only in Western medicine might rightfully say that he, too, would have come to the same conclusion, even without the Ayurvedic training. Fair enough, but that depends on a patient's being forthright about all of the things that are bothering them and self-aware enough to know that there's a problem in the first place. I can't tell you how many people are living with constipation and don't realize it. The discomfort arises gradually and becomes normalized. Listening to Mary's story was a teaching moment for me. It reinforced how important it is to ask questions and to use my Ayurvedic training in my practice. This does not mean that I practice Ayurveda; it means that I recognize the interconnectedness of the body enough to ask a patient complaining of poor sleep and headaches, "Hey, how are your bowel movements?"

This is the nexus of where my Ayurvedic training meets my Western medicine bona fides: seeing symptoms for both what they are and what they might imply; taking everything into account and thinking critically and expansively. What happens when we continually peel away at the symptoms is that we approach a problem that's multifactorial—meaning it has multiple causes—and we need to respond to it in a multifactorial way. I think you'd agree that it makes much more sense to approach each issue with a solution tailored to it. Because the other option, which a lot of doctors choose, is to throw a prescription at the problem. Can't sleep? Here are some sleeping pills. No matter that they make your rest fitful and have you slogging through the next day in a postpharmaceutical haze—sleeping pills fix sleep! I'm being facetious, of course. The multifactorial approach takes more time, but the results are more effective and lasting. And in going through the process, you learn more about yourself.

And, hell, if all else fails, of course a prescription is available!

Are Your Hot Flashes Under Control?

Why it's so important: As I mentioned earlier, hot flashes can wake you up in the middle of the night as night sweats, so frequent or out-of-control flashing can be a big sleep killer. The thing is, hot flashes are anxiety producing unto themselves, especially for those who are getting bad ones. And some of the physical effects of hot flashes are identical to those of anxiety: heart racing, feeling suffocated, uncontrolled sweating. Given all this, it's no wonder that hot flashes can take over your mind: Are you going to get hit with one right as you pipe up in a big companywide meeting? Do you feel on the verge of flashing when you're having a disagreement with your partner? How can you excuse yourself from yoga class to get some air without drawing attention to yourself? Would it be inappropriate to pull out a handheld fan during your daughter's wedding vows?

As I talked about in the previous section, hot flashes cause anxiety and are provoked by anxiety. Anxiety can spill over into depression. Therefore, managing hot flashes can be a big boon for your mental health. To give you some perspective, associating anxiety with hot flashes has been controversial, but an unusually long-term follow-up study from the University of Pennsylvania demonstrated a statistically significant relationship specifically between the so-called somatic, or body-based, symptoms of anxiety (face flushing and heart pounding) and the later experience of hot flashes during and after menopause, meaning that if your premenopausal self got worked up about something and you felt your heart go *thump thump thump* really hard in your chest, there's a higher chance that hot flashes will be part of your menopause journey. The more mood-based symptoms of anxiety—basically the emotional part without the physical manifestations—were *not* associated with the severity of hot flashes. This not only suggests a possible common cause of the body-based symptoms of anxiety and hot flashes but may have predictive value and create an opportunity for early intervention and prevention of suffering.

Addressing both the mental and physical aspects is important, and the way you should do it is unique to you. Moreover, you may need to think out of the box to find what works best for you; teasing out the "mind" part of the mind-body connection is so personal. For instance, a paper in *Menopause* reported on a group of 187 postmenopausal women who were flashing at least fifty times a week and who received five weekly sessions of either clinical hypnosis or a control activity based around attention. That went on for twelve weeks. Those in the hypnosis group saw an almost 75 percent reduction in their hot flashes, while the control group stopped at around 17 percent of their flashes. And a study from King's College London suggested that cognitive behavioral therapy—a type of therapy that teaches people how to adjust their negative thinking in a way that helps improve their behavior patterns—can work in as little as six weeks. Yes, these are small, short-term studies, but the interventions *had no dangerous side effects.*

You Don't Have "Reproductive Hormones"; You Have Hormones

Built into the training to be an ob-gyn—and really all of medical training—is the blanket assumption that every woman wants to have children and her fertility should be protected at all costs. That (a) is not true, (b) reduces women's beings to baby-making factories, and

(c) contributes to our gendered thinking about binaries. This is why I no longer refer to estrogen, progesterone, and testosterone as "reproductive hormones." Likewise, I no longer talk about reproductive organs.

On a practical level, we know that the so-called reproductive hormones and organs do more than just facilitate pregnancy. We've already discussed the incredible roles estrogen plays that go far beyond the menstrual cycle and pregnancy. It is intimately related to cognition, bone health, skin function, metabolism, and more. That makes sense, as hormones are chemical messengers connecting the brain and other hormone-producing organs to the rest of the body.

But what about the so-called reproductive organs? They certainly have one function: making babies. I mean, the alternate name of the uterus is a womb, which is expressly a home for a fetus. Medicine's preconceptions about even those organs are changing. A landmark 2018 study suggested that the uterus is a cognitive hotspot. The researchers, from Arizona State University, were interested in the effects of hysterectomy, or the removal of the uterus. They found that one-third of women have a hysterectomy by age sixty, and most of them happen before the menopausal transition. In about half of the surgeries, the ovaries are left in the body; the other half of the patients have their ovaries removed, which puts them into what's called *surgical menopause* immediately.

"The dogma is that the nonpregnant uterus is dormant," the study authors wrote. So they decided to put some unsuspecting rats through different variations of the surgery to see how it affected their memory. "Rats without ovaries learned the working memory domain of a complex cognitive task"—a test of the rat's brainpower—"faster than did those with ovaries. Moreover, uterus removal alone had a unique detrimental impact on the ability to handle a high-demand working memory load." If you recall from the previous section, we know that estrogen seems to help with brain function, which is why the loss of the hormone that occurs during menopause is associated with dementia and Alzheimer's disease. So it would be logical to assume that doing a hysterectomy but leaving the ovaries alone would be better, brainwise. But this study—albeit in rats—suggests that that might not be the case.

The study authors, writing in the journal *Endocrinology*, summed up by saying that we need to study further how the uterus and ovaries affect brain and endocrine aging, especially given how often gynecological surgeries are performed. "Moreover, findings demonstrate that *the nonpregnant uterus is not dormant*, and indicate that there is an ovarian-uterus-brain system that becomes interrupted when the reproductive tract has been disrupted, leading to alterations in brain functioning." (Emphasis mine.)

Are You Moving?

There are very few cure-alls in my business, but body movement is one of them. We already covered all the ways in which exercise is a boon for physical health. There are also reams of research showing that exercise and other physical activity is good for mental health. They increase our feeling of self-worth and make us feel more positive, which can help improve our quality of life. In the near term, movement can reduce some of the unpleasant menopause symptoms, such as hot flashes and low libido, that can contribute to anxiety and depression. Plus, exercise releases feel-good endorphins, which is why you so often walk out of an exercise class with a smile on your face. (The camaraderie of a group and the connection with a trainer or fellow gym patrons help, too.) In the long term, it can help us retain our cognitive function and remain socially connected to our community.

Medicine Has an Ableism Problem

When the medical community talks about exercise, it is speaking to those who are not living with a disability at the expense of those who are. It is ableist—meaning discriminatory in favor of people not living with disabilities—and we do not yet have the sensitivity to acknowledge equally the experience of everyone going through menopause. For people who are living in bodies that have different capabilities, I would say that body movement is helpful to the extent that you are able to do it comfortably. I think about the work of Sabrina Cohen in Miami. A C5 quadriplegic as the result of a spinal cord injury due to a car accident in 1992 at the age of fourteen, Sabrina has used the help of personal trainers educated in helping people with disabilities do strength and endurance training. One of the missions of the Sabrina Cohen Foundation is to make beaches in Miami accessible to people who have different mobility, including laying foam tracks across the sand and supplying floating chairs that allow people to be immersed in the ocean with the help of volunteers who are not disabled.

I bring up Sabrina's story because she has talked about how finding exercise that is right for her has improved her life immensely in terms of both her physical abilities and her mental health. She found people with the right expertise who could guide her along her fitness journey. And she worked really hard at it, taking a long view of progress that has paid off.

Those of us who do not use adaptive tools should not feel bad about that. We should feel bad that we live in a world that makes able-bodiedness both the ideal and the default. Being part of the push for greater inclusion and accessibility in our physical spaces, as well as ensuring that people with disabilities are not discriminated against in the workplace, in social situations, and even in medicine, is our assignment.

Exercise comes in an incredible number of forms. Along with

that, I want to clear up a misconception: exercising and moving your body do not have to be strenuous for you to get positive results from them. There are advantages to different types of exercise, but going for a walk every day, doing some stretching, scaling a couple flights of stairs—everything adds up to make a positive impact. Research from the Pennsylvania State University found that after four months of a walking or yoga program, participants who were going through the menopausal transition improved their self-reported quality of life, compared with those who did neither. Those in the walking group saw a bigger increase in their health and the emotional quality of their life, and the yogis saw an improvement in the quality of their sexual life.

I know from my personal experience, as well as that of my friends and patients, that those who make body movement a habit are better able to weather the ups and downs of menopause—and life. You can chalk this up to a lot of things: the release of feel-good endorphins that happens when we exercise; the ability to say "yes" to activities such as hiking, playing sports, frolicking in the ocean. Having these sorts of experiences is great for mental health, but we can do them only when we're physically able to.

The Power of Nature

I'm all for a bougie gym with eucalyptus towels, but if you're moving your body specifically for the mental health benefits, it's hard to beat the great outdoors. Have you heard of forest bathing? It originated in 1982 in Japan, where it is known as *shinrin-yoku*, or "taking in the forest atmosphere." A small study published in the Japanese journal *Environmental Health and Preventive Medicine* took two groups of people on either a walk in the forest or a walk in the city for fifteen minutes. The following day, the two groups flipped and did the other walk. The researchers used a few measurements: salivary cortisol (a stress hormone found in the saliva), blood pressure, pulse rate, and heart rate variability. "The results show that forest environments promote lower concentrations of cortisol, lower pulse rate, lower blood pressure, greater parasympathetic nerve activity"—which kicks in when the body is resting and relaxing—"and lower sympathetic nerve activity [the system that hypes you up] than do city environments," the study authors wrote. A study done several years later, also in Japan, involving 585 participants in their twenties walking in a forest for fifteen minutes, asked them to self-assess how they were feeling. The forest bathers reported lowered feelings of "'depression-dejection,' 'tension-anxiety,' 'anger-hostility,' 'fatigue,' and 'confusion' and improved the participants' positive mood of 'vigor' compared with walking through city areas." There's even more research showing that spending time among trees boosts the immune system, improves blood glucose levels among those with diabetes, may help fight cancer, can restore focus, and can help people with sleep problems get better shut-eye—especially when they forest bathe in the afternoon.

The effectiveness is not limited to forests, either. Time spent in nature makes us feel more connected with Earth and with one another. One thing that Ayurveda teaches is that as the seasons change, so should we. Our time spent sleeping lengthens in the winter and shortens in the summer, along with the nighttime hours. What we eat should reflect where we live and the produce that is in season at any given time. And our bodies want to be out in nature, taking in the sights of trees or mountains or bodies of water.

Nature has always been a big part of my life. I grew up going to summer camp in Ojai, California, and spending time at the beaches along the Santa Barbara coast in all seasons. In the past few years, I have spent more time in and around Joshua Tree National Park, due east of my home in Los Angeles. My meditation practice feels easier and deeper there. Looking across the landscape is itself a meditation.

I can feel in my body how the soundtrack of the desert helps slow my breathing and my heart rate. There may be hard science in respected journals saying so, but you need only spend a little time in nature to understand how powerfully connected we humans are to it.

Having access to nature is a form of privilege, and the amount of greenness available to Americans falls sharply along economic and racial lines. And historically, outdoor sports have been segregated. Women have not always been welcome in outdoor spaces, and Black women have been particularly disenfranchised; if you'd like more information about an organization that promotes walking for healing, check out GirlTrek (https://www.girltrek.org/).

Accessibility is a problem, but it is not an unsolvable one. A tree on your street that you can see from your window is grounding to look at and can create a healing experience. Growing medicinal herbs or teas, such as cilantro, lemon balm, chamomile, or lavender, connects us to nature and yields natural interventions. A small backyard vegetable garden or indoor hydroponic or window sill set-up can feel miraculous when you're watching your food grow and it comes time to harvest. I can tell you from personal experience that growing some of our food and medicinal herbs during the pandemic and the death of my mom has been the single most powerful healing factor in these last two truly challenging years.

If reading this bums you out because you feel as though you've fallen behind on exercise, let me assure you that, for starters, you're not alone. It's an unfortunate fact that women end up playing the role of caretakers to everyone around them—both at home and at work—and we're expected to use whatever's in our tanks for others. Self-care, including exercise, falls by the wayside. The timing of the menopausal transition often coincides with the transition of your kids to increased independence. It's hard to make the switch to self-care, partly because you still don't have a lot of time to yourself and also because you've been conditioned since childhood to put yourself last.

But I'm telling you, you can do it. Your first act doesn't need to be signing up for a 5:00 a.m. hot yoga class, either. Set a timer for fifteen minutes, throw on some music, and dance around; do jumping jacks and push-ups (on a chair or piece of sturdy furniture if you need to). For years, my go-to was the famous *New York Times* seven-minute scientific workout! But your activity doesn't have to be that newsy. Meet a friend for a walk in a park. Ride your bike to do errands instead of driving your car; getting your exercise in and reducing your carbon footprint at the same time is a win-win.

We'll get more into the specifics of exercise for your postmenopause life in the final part of the book, but I want to mention one more thing: your body will respond to exercise the moment you start doing it. Take exercise's effect on your brain; a study in *Journal of Aging and Physical Activity* published in 2010 found that healthy older adults who went for a twenty-minute walk had greater cognitive processing speed than those who sat quietly for the same amount of time. Interested in improving your blood pressure? Even one session of weight training can help do that, and lifting weights on a consistent basis can have lasting effects, according to research published in *European Journal of Applied Physiology*. Speaking of lasting effects, a review of research published in *Exercise and Sport Sciences Reviews* found that exercise might have an even more pronounced ability to reduce breast cancer risk among postmenopausal people versus those who are premenopausal.

Are You Feeling More Forgetful than Usual?

This is a big thing that people start to feel down about. It automatically makes you feel old. Forgetfulness happens. It's extremely common, with more than half of women reporting it. An interesting study from Australia published in the journal *Climacteric* in 2010 found that among a group of 120 women, 79 percent of those who were in peri-menopause reported attention problems and 82 percent had memory problems. Compare that with the postmenopausal women: 68 percent had attention problems, and 79 percent had memory problems. Which means that even if you're searching for words and forgetting why you went to the grocery store now, things could get better. (Useful to know, too: among premenopausal women, half reported attention problems and 77 percent memory problems—so maybe we all need to give our brains some TLC.) The study authors said that the subjective and objective data they'd gathered supports what people describe as feeling "cloudiness" or "blocking" when it comes to their thinking processes. The sudden loss of short-term memory affects brain function; we know that diminished sleep and hot flashes are contributors. We also know that memory issues can cause mood issues. So again, this is a complex chain of events that has some biological components and some mental components, and where one ends and the other begins is anyone's guess at this point.

But here's the rub: our cognitive abilities go hand in hand with factors such as stress. Whether we're menopausal or not, the more stressed out we are, the worse our brains are going to work. And, you guessed it: sleep is essential. Skimping on sleep is a surefire way to send your memory and thought processing straight to the trash compactor.

We also know that stress is a drag on memory and that some populations are more susceptible to chronic stress. For instance, a study found that low-income women of color, some of whom were HIV positive, had longer-lasting cognitive declines going into postmenopause. The study, published in *Menopause*, said that it could be because of risk factors such as less education, a history of trauma, mental health issues, and HIV or hepatitis C infection status.

But there are things that can be done about it. A review of research conducted at Baylor University in Waco, Texas, sought to investigate the mind-body part of memory decline. They found several small studies in which practicing yoga and mindfulness had helped with hot flashes (they also help improve sleep, which is a big factor in cognition). One small study that looked at yoga versus general exercise for cognitive performance found that both help with memory but yoga helped women more.

Eating a healthy diet and cutting out drinking are two ways to improve your cognitive function. If you've ever been hungover from a night of drinking, you know that the brain is in a bad way. Alcohol is a depressant and slows down communication between neurons. And it dehydrates the body, which the brain does not enjoy. Try to stock your refrigerator with loads of fruits and vegetables—whether frozen or fresh, they have the same nutritional value. Focus on berries for their flavonoids and antioxidants, which have myriad powers including promoting memory and cognitive function. The vitamins and antioxidants in leafy greens may help slow cognitive decline, too.

Do You Have a Support System at Home and at Work?

As I mentioned previously, there's an epidemic of loneliness in the United States, especially among older adults. According to the National Institute on Aging (NIA), "Research has linked social isolation and loneliness to higher risks for a variety of physical and mental conditions: high blood pressure, heart disease, obesity, a weakened immune system, anxiety, depression, cognitive decline, Alzheimer's disease, and even death." You could argue that these are the risk factors that arise from being older. And it strikes me, reading through this list, how much overlap there is with the risks associated with being postmenopausal. To understand this, it's important to consider the words "risk factor." Each risk factor has a magnifying effect on the others. And you can't help the fact that you're aging, nor can you control your menopause status. But you *do* have agency over your lifestyle. And, like body movement, connection with others is a cure-all.

"People who engage in meaningful, productive activities with others tend to live longer, boost their mood, and have a sense of purpose," the NIA says. "These activities seem to help maintain their well-being and may improve their cognitive function, studies show." It's the *with others* part that is important. You probably feel it, too: the feel-good power of being around people who make you feel supported and share your interests.

We're not just talking about sewing circles and book clubs. Increasingly, we have to accept that work is a place where menopause happens. Though the covid-19 pandemic pushed a lot of women out of the workforce, overall, middle-aged and older people are staying in the workforce for longer as the retirement age is pushed back. And the timing of the menopausal transition means that women may be hitting their stride at work concurrently. A paper written by three members of the Faculty of Medicine and Health at the University of Sydney in Australia argued that if workplaces want to retain age diversification and expertise, they need to be mindful of menopause—even consider it an occupational safety issue, especially related to hot flashes. In fact, other research coming out of the United Kingdom found that "menopausal status was not associated with work outcomes but having problematic hot flushes at work was associated with intention to stop working." Loss of work can equal a loss of purpose and fulfillment. It can also cause financial insecurity, which is a huge stressor that itself has downstream effects, such as our old friend the hot flash. It's a reality that people find purpose and camaraderie at work, as well as financial security.

When I say a support system, it includes your place of employment. What if offices had cooling rooms for menopausal people as they do lactation areas for breastfeeding? What if you could be candid with your supervisor, regardless of their gender or age, about why your work product has been a little off lately or that you are having back-to-back headaches or things are slipping your mind more than usual? What if you could feel empowered to get up and leave a meeting if you experienced a sudden and unexpectedly heavy menstrual bleeding episode? What if you could rely on coworkers to help you out when you need a breather? To some people, this sounds like pie in the sky, and if you work in Silicon Valley, a notoriously misogynistic tech haven, you may have closed this book and chucked it across the room. *But this is what progress would look like!* Listen, I work in a private ob-gyn practice, and even I don't feel as though this is immediately within reach.

I get a little more hopeful when I see what's happening in the United Kingdom. In 2017, its Department for Education commissioned a study on the economic contribution that menopausal women make. It found that the fastest-growing demographic in the workforce is menopausal women, and around 80 percent of menopausal women are employed. With such a large percentage of menopausal people experiencing symptoms, it's incumbent on employers to create a more inclusive and responsive workplace for them. Organizations including the British national television network Channel 4 have been out front on the subject. Some policies being adopted include designating cool spaces for use during hot flashes, recognizing the necessity for menstrual leave, and opening dialogues to destigmatize menopause.

I hope this is the direction US workplaces are going in. If this essential component of the workforce is to be kept at companies, *in the workforce at all*, changes need to happen. In the meantime, think about ways you can be a support system for others who need it. If you have an opportunity to have candid conversations about what you're experiencing, it opens the door for other people to share their stories if they choose. If you're feeling a bit like Norma Rae, you could even press your company's leadership to make menopause-friendly changes.

What Do We Lose When We Are
Reduced to Our Hormones?

During the course of my twenty-five-plus-year career, our knowledge about hormones has grown. While reading about how complex the hormonal feedback loops are and how many of them exist, you may wonder: Are we simply the sum of our hormones?

Short answer: No, we are way more than our hormones. All of the books that tell you that you need to get your hormones under control are looking at things the wrong way. The books that tell you that you'd better wrangle those hormones to the floor if you ever want to lose weight and be sexually desirable again—well, those books can go to hell. Your hormones are fluctuating. If it makes sense for you and you choose to, going on menopausal hormone therapy can be a way for you to compensate for the chemical changes that are happening in your body. Is MHT the be-all and end-all that'll make you feel as though you're twenty-five again? No. You still need to be vigilant about your physical and mental health.

Maybe you're thinking that I'm contradicting myself. After all, we've covered the fact that many of the symptoms of menopause are driven largely by fluctuating hormones that are undergoing a sudden downward adjustment. And hormonal changes beget other hormonal changes. Hormones are the chemical messengers that control our desires for things such as sleep, sex, affection, and food. Hormones are behind losing hair on our heads and gaining it on our faces, how well our bones repair, and the energy we have to go about our day. These changes can manifest themselves in hot flashes and out-of-control PMS-like symptoms.

What I want to remind you is that the timing of these changes is important. You may be transitioning from parenting younger children to older ones, which requires a rethinking of your role in the family structure. Perhaps work is hitting its stride and you're rising in the ranks and owning your career—or maybe you're heading for a career pivot. And the physical changes you're noticing in your body, both the way you feel in it and its outward appearance, are bringing up some uncomfortable feelings.

So I can give you menopausal hormone therapy and it might ameliorate a bunch of physical symptoms. But that doesn't take the place of your doing work on yourself, exploring what's going on between your ears—especially with the help of a professional. If you're resistant to that and want everything to just be *fixed*, I fear you'll end up disappointed. If you haven't yet done so, it's time to stop fighting your body. Learning to live with your genetic code, your hormonal fluctuations, your appearance, and the way your body feels *and finding peace* is the only way to have peace. Living in the shadow of shame is no way to live. I know that's reductive, but it's hard to have happiness and fulfilment without also having peace and owning your authentic existence.

Do You Practice Self-Care?

If the answer is "I don't," you've got some work to do! But don't feel bad if that is your answer. In the binary female-male world most of us grew up in, girls were groomed to be caretakers, and our jobs included putting the needs of others above our own. This is the work of the patriarchy, which created a system in which men are the doers and women are the supporters. It infuriates me. So you've spent the better part of four decades giving out energy to the people around you. But how much have you been receiving in return? The equation is probably lopsided.

That dynamic's been happening forever. What gives me chills is what passes these days for self-care. I know that the covid-19 pandemic has been horrible for women in particular. They've had to shoulder the burden of homeschooling and running a household in a home that was not made to house everyone full-time in a warped kind of house arrest. Many had to leave the workforce, and economists believe that this is going to set women in the workplace back many years. And there's not much time for self-care in a pandemic when your only time of solace is going to the bathroom (and only if you don't have toddlers). The self-care proxy for millions of women has been drinking. A study by the RAND Corporation revealed that heavy drinking days—defined as having four or more drinks within a few hours—among women were up by 41 percent in 2020. As a physician, I'm terrified for women's physical and mental health when I see data like these.

I'm not judging people who have responded this way. I get it. The late Dr. Henry S. Lodge, who was an excellent physician and a coauthor of the book *Younger Next Year: Live Strong, Fit, and Sexy—Until You're 80 and Beyond*, wrote about the myth of "me time." The fact is that women spend the entire day making sure the needs of others are taken care of and running themselves ragged in the process. By the time dinner has been cleaned up and the kids are in bed, they crave self-care and acknowledgment of what they've accomplished that day. "Me time" can take the form of a glass (or two) of wine with a salty or sweet snack while watching thirty minutes or an hour of television. Dr. Lodge said pointedly that they'd be better off going to bed; they could benefit from the extra sleep and certainly didn't need the wine or chips or ice cream. He was right, of course—though I'd argue that staying up a little longer to practice healthier forms of self-care is time well spent. Here's what I have in mind.

Begin a Meditation Practice

A lot of people, especially high-performing women, are afraid of meditating. They think that they're supposed to clear their minds, except that they can never clear their minds because they have too many to-do lists, unfinished home projects, and lingering fights with their mom to be able to get to a place of inner peace and calm. What I tell them is this: The goal isn't to stop thoughts from entering your brain. That's impossible. Instead, you want to observe your thoughts and try not to engage with them. Some people say that thoughts are like bubbles that float into the picture and out again. It takes practice! Start with thirty seconds once or twice a day. Then increase it to one minute, two minutes, and keep adding on until you get to about thirty minutes. There are a lot of apps and accessories out there to help you, and there's just tons of great research about all of the ways meditation helps you, specifically during menopause. Research published in 2019 by the Menopause & Women's Sexual Health Clinic at Mayo Clinic in Rochester found that midlife women who scored higher on a mindfulness scale and had lower stress reported less severe menopausal symptoms. Plus, practicing mindfulness may help reduce resting cortisol levels, found researchers at the UC Davis Center for Mind and Brain. And higher cortisol levels are associated with problems such as accumulation of belly fat and cardiac issues.

So seriously, please start meditating. If this is new territory for you, find an app that can lead you through visualizations and give you time cues, based on what you want to achieve during your session, your experience, and the time you want to spend. Headspace and Calm are two popular ones. In-person meditation classes are great, too. You might find one in a meditation or complementary medicine center or a yoga studio. The lotus pose (padmasana) is the traditional position for meditation; it's done seated on the ground, your legs crossed in front of you and the toes of each foot on top of the opposite knee. If you do not have the flexibility to do this pose, use a pillow or bolster under your butt to take pressure off your hips and knees. If it's hard on your back, a meditation chair might be the ticket. But honestly, the pose isn't the important part. Sitting in a chair is fine! Ideally, some part of your body—possibly the bottoms of your feet—

will make contact with the ground. The object isn't to be comfortable but to be engaged.

I've been practicing meditation for about twenty years. Some days focus comes easily, some days not. That's why it's referred to as a *practice*. People think they should be good at it, and if their minds don't clear away the clutter on demand as though Marie Kondo is on their brain's speed dial, the practice is somehow not for them. One thing that can help get you into the zone is creating a ritual around meditation. Mine involves the meditation table that sits in my bedroom. It's small—around two feet square—and sits close to the ground. It's an unobtrusive constant in my sight line when I'm in my bedroom, coaxing me to my meditation practice when I'm ready for it. You'll find these in the homes of many people who practice Ayurveda. It is covered in objects that have meaning for me. Its presence is like a cocoon of calm and a reminder that I am loved by others, myself, and the universe. That's how I feel when my eyes fall on the mala beads that were a gift from a dear friend; small stones and shells picked up on local walks and faraway travels; homemade art by my kids; a turkey feather a friend found on a hike, which carried symbolism that made her think of me. Sometimes I add an object to help me manifest something I'm desiring. Other times an object has served its purpose and I remove it. The table has a little card on it, folded up, that I placed there on the first of the year. Every New Year's Eve, I write one with my intentions for the next twelve months, and those scribblings act to center me when I leave the path and start metaphorically bushwhacking in unhelpful ways. (Helpful bushwhacking is encouraged.)

Find Your Flow State

In the past couple years, it seems as though the ranks of people who either knit or made pottery just about tripled. I suspect it's because those are among the activities that put you into what is called a flow state. This is when your brain stops thinking, yet your body is still calmly active. There's a bit of muscle memory involved. Repetitive activity is a big part of achieving a flow state. Sometimes it's achieved for minutes at a time, sometimes seconds. Even if you've never identified a flow state in your life, I'd bet you've experienced it. While going for a run, for example, there are periods where it feels as though you're on autopilot and your brain is not registering discomfort or calculating how long you have to go. That's a flow state. If you play tennis and enter into a long rally with your opponent or hitting partner, you feel as though you can anticipate where each ball will land, and it bounces off the middle of your racquet perfectly every time: that's a flow state. (Unsurprisingly, athletes often chase flow states.) It can even happen when you're driving on the highway and you're feeling really connected to the road and calm; you're in a flow state. Now, if some jerk cuts you off and you swerve or have to slam on the brakes, they've both endangered you and broken your flow state.

Do you have an activity that puts you into a flow state? I find delight and surprise in the flow states that occur when I least expect them: during a mediation or a workout or at home when I am cooking or gardening.

Pick a Mantra

If you're worried about your racing mind, pick a mantra to repeat during your practice. Sit in a comfortable position, your legs crossed if it feels natural to you, your eyes closed, feeling the connection between your body and the ground. Borrow my mantra (which is itself borrowed from the brilliant Metta Loving-Kindness Meditation instructor George Haas) until you come up with your own: "I love you. Keep going." Direct that to yourself.

Find Your Way to a Yoga Mat

This goes hand in hand with meditation. In fact, it's traditionally used to prepare the mind and body for meditation. I think that yoga is outstanding for a few reasons: It works on balance and flexibility and is weight bearing, both of which help with injury prevention. It gets your blood flowing. If you have insomnia, it seems to help with sleep. It builds body positivity, self-awareness, and self-confidence. Yoga is practical movement that asks you to go from the ground to standing and works the small muscles in the lower body that keep you steady on your feet. But more than its practical components, yoga teaches us that we are connected to the earth and with one another. And I like how yoga talks about goals. We should strive to become comfortable with discomfort and not to panic in the face of pain or challenge. Yoga teaches us that failure comes from not trying, rather than trying and not succeeding.

Give Yourself Self-Massage and Oil Treatments

Ayurveda teaches us the importance of daily self-massage (no, not that kind, but that is also more than acceptable). Some of the benefits include improvements in blood circulation, skin, muscle, and joint tone and texture, as well as better sleep and mood. Touch induces the release of hormones associated with feelings of love. More recent research indicates that touch activates the parasympathetic nervous system. And regulating the stress response is a benefit of any kind of massage. Some studies have looked at how massage can contribute to many types of recovery, including from stroke and addiction. If you don't already practice self-massage, try adding it to your self-care activities. It is a traditional method of healing, but I have modified it and teach it in this way.

Dedicate the last ninety seconds of your shower to self-massage. Use an organic oil of your choice. Sesame is the traditional base oil, but it can be a bit smelly, so I often opt for safflower, grapeseed, or coconut oil. Add a few drops of an aromatherapy oil. For instance, rose oil or lavender is used to bring calm, clary sage to cool, citrus to energize and elevate mood, and rosemary or oregano to boost immunity. Working from head to toes and from periphery to torso, apply and massage the oil into warm, wet skin in long strokes on the long parts and in circular motions over joints. Do the same over your breasts, butt, and abdomen. Follow the course of your large intestines from your right lower quadrant up across the top of the belly and down to the left, or descending, colon. The oil is very slippery, so be careful to stand on a towel or slip-resistant mat. And if the towel gets soaked in oil, *do not dry it in the dryer*. You may light your house on fire!

Try or Continue Journaling or Writing

I've been a writer for as long as I can remember, and my writing expresses itself in different ways depending on where I am in my life. Sometimes it's related to a specific thing I'm going through, or I keep a dream journal. I also use medicine cards, authored by an Indigenous man and woman and based on southwestern Indigenous animal medicine beliefs and practices. They're akin to tarot cards, and they enable me to access deeper insights into what I'm experiencing and feeling. They never fail to help me come to an answer or reframe a decision that I hadn't thought of before. I use these cards as a touchstone.

You've gleaned from this that I don't have one singular writing practice, but I do find ways to express myself in words. I find that it helps me work through problems, and I hope that you will find ways to express yourself through writing and explore greater self-understanding, too. If writing in a journal every night is the best way for you to do that, awesome! If it feels good to write mantras that you can call upon during a yoga practice, while on a run, or in your everyday life, that's incredible. There's no one thing that is the best. One caveat: I'm a big proponent of writing on paper versus typing on a computer or your phone. There's something powerful about the tactile experience and seeing your own handwriting. And for me, writing forces me to slow down. My fingers can type faster than my brain can think, and that delay can give me the impression that I'm stuck or that a problem is intractable. Usually, though, I'm not stuck; I just need to give my mind a little more time.

CHAPTER 6

Menopause and Mood Disorders

I talked earlier about how depression and anxiety are multifactorial, and once you start peeling away the layers, you can start to unearth the core issues for *you*. NIH researchers sought to discover the prevalence of mood disorders, so they followed twenty-nine premenopausal women until they'd gone six months without having a period. Nine women became depressed during the course of the study, and six of them hadn't had depressive episodes before. "For the 24 months surrounding the final menses, the risk for onset of depression was 14 times as high as for a 31-year premenopausal period of time," the researchers found—meaning that if you find yourself in this boat, there are millions of other passengers in it with you.

Help via a professional therapist is more accessible than ever with telemedicine. For some people, medication helps, whether it's for mental health or to address hormone replacement. Finding a community helps. Having conversations with people who understand what you're going through and people who don't understand firsthand but want to understand your experience better—that also helps.

Create Spaces That Reflect Who You Are

I was having a Zoom call with Mona Eltahawy, who's an incredible writer, speaker, and thinker who focuses on Arab and Muslim issues and global feminism. Hanging above her couch was a painting of a woman, nude from the waist up, arms outstretched, head tilted up, and red-lipsticked mouth yelling out. Across her chest and torso was written THERE WILL BE MILLIONS OF US. The painting, by the Indigenous artist Nadine Faraj, is an homage to Amina Sboui, also known as Amina Tyler. She is the Tunisian feminist who, on March 11, 2013, at age nineteen, posted a topless photo on Facebook. Written in Arabic across her body was "Fuck your morals. My body belongs to me and is not the source of anyone's honor." Religious zealots called for her to be lashed and stoned to death. She was eventually arrested and sent to prison for vandalism and other charges. The phrase worn by the woman in the painting relays that the movement does not start and end with Amina Tyler, and it is not contained by geography, either. There are people who are willing to stand up for body autonomy the world over, even when the cost of their courage and conviction is steep.

The painting, which Eltahawy looks at every day, is sheer power. It's a physical object that embodies the phrase "Death to the patriarchy." Given the work that Eltahawy does, I imagine there are days when it all feels very heavy. That painting is energy. And I imagine it's not a coincidence that this is where she conducts video chats for work. In my own office, the painting behind my desk, which patients see in the background of our conversations—in person or on video chat—is an abstract interpretation of a nude figure, neither female nor male. The vibrant colors and boldness catch the eye and invite curiosity. People comment on it a lot. My hope is to say something about myself and our interaction through this artwork: that I am open to you as you are; that I have energy to give and invite you to bring your energy to this place; that I am not a stodgy old doctor and you don't have to edit yourself around me.

Come to my home, and there's a different vibe. I need a place that imparts calm. It was a conscious decision I made in 2008, the year I remodeled the house, which I had already lived in for the previous eleven years. When my ex-husband moved out, I changed the art and the furniture. The remodeled house is one my ex never lived in. This space would see my children through the rest of their childhood and would eventually create a life including a man named Greg. His entrance into our lives—and the addition of three cats—transformed the house even more. Greg broke ground on the garden out back. It has been his project. It is a literal way to "ground" ourselves in this new place, which is the foundation of our growing life together. Throughout all of the changes, I have been conscious about creating a space that represents who I am and who I want to be and the family I am part of.

Like so many other people, in earlier years, I wanted to hide certain parts of myself and project others that might not be so true. You don't need to conceal yourself. It's only when we bring that deep-down part of ourselves to the surface and beyond that we can live our most authentic lives. It's difficult, but if you haven't done it yet, the menopausal transition is—I've got to tell you—the perfect time. Our bodies are demanding self-discovery, and our minds are demanding reflection.

Do you have touchstones around you that feel like a physical representation of who you are and what's important to you? Put them front and center. Draw from them the energy you need. Like the healing crystals that we imbue with the qualities we want—calm, clarity, wisdom, lightheartedness—having these reminders can be grounding. They become even more important during a time when so many of us are feeling the earth shaking below our feet.

Reexamine Your Relationship with Time

I grew up in a family that valued service. Making contributions to the people and world around you gives life meaning, or so I learned from my liberal doctor dad and classic stay-at-home 1970s turned Renaissance woman mom. They weren't wrong, but in learning that lesson, I picked up a bad habit: assuming that if the people around me weren't always actively pursuing something, if they seemed to be operating at a slower pace or took a pause, that they were not operating at the same level as go-getters like me. Probably it's not a coincidence that my partner, Greg, has a similar work ethic. On a Saturday morning when I'm catching extra zzz's after a long workweek, I'll often hear the lawn mower zooming around the yard, pushed by Greg, who's already been up for a couple hours. And he, like me, has done a full week in a job that's physically taxing. Now, I'm not saying I don't like going downstairs to a clean kitchen and a weeded front walkway, but I fear his father's and grandfather's disdain for idling rubbed off on him.

Now that I'm in my fifties, I realize that I cannot operate at the same breakneck speed I have always expected of myself. Of course, the fact that I have a choice about this is evidence of my privilege. Not everyone can choose to pull back. Maybe you are working more than one job or are caring for parents or children with special needs. For you, the idea of pulling back may be unfathomable. I feel for you. And I hope there will come a day when your burden eases. But I've begun to think about the Jewish tradition of Shabbat. I'm not an observant

Jew, so I don't prohibit myself from working, driving a car, purchasing things, and the like on that day. However, the time set aside to rest and reflect speaks to me. Observant Jews use this time to pray and think about their relationship with God and the people around them. My Shabbat is an opportunity to reconnect with my spiritual side, which doesn't get much attention during the week. The oil massage I do in the shower lasts a little longer, a sign that I am engaging in greater self-care. And I use this rest as a way to quiet all of the noise in my life and find the voices that I can't hear over the din. While doing so, I might realize that I haven't spoken to a friend in a while, one who's going through a tough time, and drop her a note. Perhaps I haven't volunteered in a while and make a plan to recommit. Or I realize that the most recent conversation I had with a family member ended on a slightly sour note, and I give them a call to resolve it.

I know what you're thinking: "Good for you that you can have your me time on a weekend. But have you seen my Google calendar and inbox lately? Do you *know* how many damn baked goods the PTA expects me to bake?" Yes, I get it. And without sounding like your out-of-touch friend, gliding into your living room wearing a caftan and smelling like sandalwood (all of which could absolutely happen if we were friends), the hard truth is that you just have to make time. Take ownership of your time. It's part of being a grown-up at this point in your life. You're probably going to disappoint some people in the process. Maybe your workplace, like mine, expects you to be available via email and phone at whatever time of the day or night. Or you have a reputation for being a superparent/spouse/friend and people depend on you. Start by setting small boundaries. Scan emails once when you get home from work, and respond only if it's truly necessary. Carve out two hours of time on the weekend for yourself; not to do errands or clean out your closet (unless those things bring you joy, of course). The PTA will earn just as much from break-and-bake cookies as it does from ones made from scratch.

Reimagining your relationship with time is deceptively hard. Here's the thought process that kept me from doing it for so long: My standing as a parent, a life partner, a doctor, and a work partner relies on the time and effort I devote to those identities. If I want to reclaim some time, it's going to have to come from somewhere. And when I do so, I'm going to end up disappointing people. I was not willing to accept that calculation for a long time and instead fulfilled all my roles. Eventually, life forced the issue. Life finds a way! My marriage fell apart, breast cancer happened, and the menopausal transition started. At a certain point I had to grow up and own my shit. I couldn't give all of myself anymore, and I didn't want to.

I'd like to tell you that I didn't disappoint people along the way. And doing so set off siren alarms in my head. It made me feel terrible to disappoint colleagues and loved ones, and it really screwed with my identity. *If Suzanne is not an exceptional parent/life partner/doctor/ work partner, then who is she?* I don't know the answer to that. I've just nibbled at the corners of scaling back. Not delivering babies in order to protect my sleep was one big step. Celebrating my children's growing independence instead of fretting over it was another. I don't know that evolutionary biology has an explanation for why the menopausal transition sets all this off in many of us, but I'm leaning in to it.

If you're not convinced, let me try one more tack. The pandemic has made two things abundantly clear: the burnout that we're all on the precipice (or deep in the depths) of and the fact that capitalism is built on the free labor of women and people of color, in addition to the disproportionately small compensation that those people—and *especially* women of color—receive compared with White people and White men in particular. (If you want more information about this, I highly recommend checking out the Nap Ministry at https://thenapministry .wordpress.com, which convincingly argues that rest is resistance and that removing yourself at times from a system that demands that you sacrifice your energy to keep it going is a way to dismantle capitalism and the patriarchy and aid the social justice movement.)

As I said, I recognize how much privilege I have. I have multiple income streams: I have my medical practice, I am part of a startup, and I wrote this book. My kids are off at college and don't have to worry about loans. I am a partner in my medical practice, which gives me more autonomy. I do not live with disabilities, nor does Greg or my children. I'm a cis White lady living in SoCal. But I hope you will know I'm genuine when I say that paring back my life and protecting time for myself recharges my batteries so I have more of myself to give to the things that are important to me, to fulfill the ideal of service to others that my parents instilled in me a half century ago.

CHAPTER 7

Prejudice in Medicine

> When the Medical System Doesn't Work
> For You, You Need to Work the System

Some of you will identify with the specific experiences the people I've interviewed for this book have shared. Others won't. For me, the tie that binds is this: the Menopause Bootcamp is about empowering ourselves with knowledge and solidarity so we can be better advocates for ourselves and others as we move through this transition and embrace what comes after. But there are people who have been systematically disenfranchised by the Western medical system since its inception. Many if not most of us have experienced some sort of medical-related trauma, regardless of our level of privilege. It's different for everyone, but common experiences include a doctor minimizing symptoms or fears, not respecting a birth plan, or judging a patient based on things such as gender expression or lifestyle. And we know, and are learning more and more every day, that how well you fare in a hospital is too often based on your race or gender, something I'll talk about later.

Here's where the goal of this book can feel as if it's at odds with the world we live in. Is it possible to be empowered patients, engaged in our care and advocating for ourselves—and do it in a system that undermines our voice and agency?

I am cautiously optimistic that the answer is yes.

To overcome the challenge of getting appropriate medical care no matter your race, sexual orientation, presentation, disability, or other identity that is used as a tool to "other" anyone who isn't a cisgendered, heterosexual White man, we have to understand in what ways the system fails the rest of us. Then we can make a plan to successfully navigate our own care. It's a tall order, and it won't work every time. Several people brought up Serena Williams's harrowing, near-fatal experience when giving birth to her daughter, Olympia, in 2017. Following an emergency C-section, the iconic professional tennis player was feeling short of breath. She has a history of blood clots and immediately alerted the nurse that she feared she was having a pulmonary embolism—meaning that blood clots were forming in a lung. The nurses pooh-poohed her, saying that she was just tired and loopy from the pain meds. Williams later said she had told the staff she needed a CT scan, and a doctor had done an ultrasound on her legs instead. "I was like, a Doppler? I told you, I need a CT scan and a heparin drip," she recalled in a 2018 *Vogue* article. Her complications didn't end there, and she had two more surgeries and spent the first six weeks at home on bed rest.

As an obstetrician, I'm horrified by what Williams went through. I am not the first to wonder what would have happened if she hadn't known her own medical history so well and then pushed the nurses to listen to her. The obvious question that follows is: If Serena Williams is not listened to, is there any hope for other women of color?

That's what the sad truth is. Black women and people of color have vastly different medical outcomes than White people do. Their maternal mortality rate is higher. White folks are more likely to be given kidney dialysis or transplants. The quality of cardiac, stroke, and cancer care and treatment for AIDS is lower for Black people. Black people are more likely to be denied pain medications or given lower dosages for myriad reasons, one of which is a racist, antebellum belief held by some health care "professionals" that Black people don't feel as much pain as White people do. (My blood is boiling as I write this.) Here's how an American Bar Association write-up of a 2005 report by the National Academy of Medicine summarized an aspect of the findings:

> Black patients with heart disease received older, cheaper, and more conservative treatments than their white counterparts. Black patients were less likely to receive coronary bypass operations and angiography. After surgery, they are discharged earlier from the hospital than white patients—at a stage when discharge is inappropriate. The same goes for other illnesses. Black women are less likely than white women to receive radiation therapy in conjunction with a mastectomy. In fact, they are less likely to receive mastectomies. Perhaps more disturbing is that black patients are *more likely* to receive *less desirable* treatments. The rates at which black patients have their limbs amputated is higher than those for white patients. Additionally, black patients suffering from bipolar disorder are more likely to be treated with antipsychotics despite evidence that these medications have long-term negative effects and are not effective.

Access to care is disproportionately lower in communities of color, especially those of Indigenous people, which means they are less likely to get preventive care, which leads to unhealthier aging and can contribute to earlier death.

There's even a menopausal connection. It appears that, on average, Black and Latina women enter menopause two years before White women do and that their menopausal transition is longer. Black and Latina women also have worse hot flashes, though the worst hot flashes are endured by Native American or Indigenous people. Socioeconomic realities and stress stemming from systemic racism contribute to this dynamic, which leads to wear and tear on the body that pushes certain women into menopause earlier. Whatever the cause, it's alarming.

My guess is that if you're a person of color or in another marginalized group, reading that will have been excruciating, but not shocking. The medical system has been coercive and abusive to communities of color. The syphilis study at Tuskegee University, which ran from 1932 to 1972 and involved leaving the syphilis of 399 Black men untreated and depriving the men of penicillin, just to see what would happen to them, is a prime example. There are other less famous but no less harrowing instances. Dr. Deirdre Cooper Owens wrote a book called *Medical Apartheid: The Dark History of Medical Experimentation on Black Americans from Colonial Times to the Present* on, among other things, the history of gynecology. For instance, "the modern father of gynecology"—whom I am intentionally not naming here—made his "discoveries" via the torture of Black enslaved women—Anarcha, Betsey, and Lucy—in the name of experimentation without anesthesia to develop now commonly used surgical techniques and instruments, including the speculum.

"The biggest challenge that women of color—especially Black women—face when it comes to aging is getting quality care from their doctors," said Denise Pines, a member of the Osteopathic Medical Board of California and a former president of the Medical Board of California. Pines is a tireless advocate for transforming the systems that exclude or punish Black women: health care, the economy, housing, technology, and public schooling, to name a few.

"Black women and other women of color are not listened to," Pines said. "So when they go to the doctor, they are already at a disadvantage. These women know this. Many times, this leads to them not returning to the doctor, and they end up suffering later in life because they delayed medical action early on."

What does it mean for a patient not to be heard?

"Doctors have a way of already making a diagnosis even before they see the patient," Pines said. "The physician reviews the chart from a medical assistant—weight, race, and ailment or what you came in for—and they already have a treatment prescribed before they even speak with you and listen to what else you may offer. They fail to really diagnose you or perform discovery tests to find out what may truly be your health challenge. So this is what every patient is up against, and if you're a woman of color, racism factors into this greatly. This can't be overstated."

Members of the Queer community, and those such as Mona Eltahawy who are both Queer and people of color, find that medicine has not made the strides to be inclusive. "The medical establishment was cis heterosexual male dominated; then cis heterosexual feminist white females entered the field," she said. "We need to push it into the rest of us: Black women; Indigenous people; women of color; Queer women. Also trans men, nonbinary people, gender nonconfirming—generally, people who have ever menstruated."

Eltahawy, sporting short-cut hair dyed the neon yellow of a tennis ball, talked about how powerful she feels now. (She's also one of the few people I've met who seems to enjoy using the F-bomb as much as I do.) It's directed to lots of things: patriarchy, classism, colonialism, ableism, homophobia, and even the idea that the transformational time that is menopause is treated like an ailment to be cured.

"I don't have anything against practitioners of medicine," she said. "But menopause is a life stage and should not be medicalized, made into a disease. It's something that happens to all of us who have or had a uterus. Inclusive language would be moving away from using the terms symptom-disease to impact-effect. This is a natural stage of life, and getting older is a celebration: I'm still here."

I recognize that as a physician, I'm a member of a profession that's behind the times. There are a lot of us who are trying to buck the trend, but it's not enough. Too many people in this country are getting inadequate care and, perhaps even worse, are made to feel invisible or othered, or it's conveyed to them that they are somehow *wrong* just because of who they are. If a doctor has ever made you feel like that, I am so sorry. I witnessed it in my training. My profession has some people who are excellent practitioners and some other not-so-great humans. That's not on you; that's on them. Please don't let that stop you from going to the doctor. Too many people delay care owing to bad experiences dealing with doctors, among other things. A delay can mean the difference between a good health outcome and a bad one.

So how do you know who's good? Ask a friend! Word of mouth is the way many of my patients come to me. I've come to learn that this is an important part of the Queer community, which has endured painful interactions with the medical system. Medical information that speaks to people across the spectrums of gender and sex can be hard to come by, so closed groups have popped up to provide support to and share experiences among people in communities that have been marginalized by medicine. Recently, I spoke with Meg Bradbury, the founder of the in-person and online group Elderqueer. The group is limited to those age forty-plus, and its programming and discussions cover the gamut of topics, including relationships, sex and dating, hormone treatments, societal forces such as capitalism and patriarchy, coming out later in life, and, of course, the menopausal transition.

"There's a comfort in queer space that's not in mixed or cis-dominant spaces," Bradbury told me. "It's a feeling of safety, community, and bravery that comes from affinity."

Transition is celebrated by Elderqueer. It's the celebration of the thing happening—the self morphing and maturing; the celebration of going through it in the warm embrace of a group of people who understand where you're at, rather than having to go through it privately or with just your partner or another couple. It's a celebration that these rites of passage are not something to be ashamed of.

"Why do I feel guilty for going through the menopausal transition?" Bradbury asked rhetorically. "Why am I made to feel I've done something wrong? Where are our stories here? We have stories for most transitions in our life, but we become less and less relevant and valid. Add 'Queer,' and then we feel even more dismissiveness."

I asked Bradbury about the Elderqueer logo. "There's wisdom, warmth, strength, and healing," she explained. "What I try to convey is older people have all of those things to impart on younger people in the community." This goes against so much of what aging people in all communities experience that spans all genders—including men: the idea that older folks are not able to keep up, have less to contribute, ought to make their way to the sidelines. It ties back to capitalism: our worth has been commodified; the less productive we are, the less value we have. Bradbury summmed it up pretty tidily: "So many things attached to the idea of being older that are just fucked."

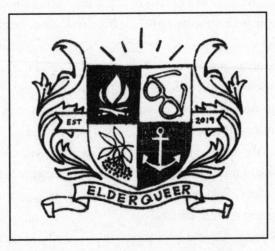

Elderqueer Crest Artwork by Kavel Rafferty

The social and psychological value of groups such as Elderqueer and the work of people such as Bradbury are invaluable. But they still can't do Pap smears. The medical system is going to have to reform in a way that invites *all* people in. It shouldn't be a patient's job to vet doctors for things like their ability to display basic human decency. I think it will always be the case that some physicians are better versed in specific issues that come up in the Queer community, but it should always be the case that patients are treated with the utmost respect and that doctors feel empowered to sometimes say, "I don't know the answer to that, but I'll research it and find out" or "I don't think I'm the best-qualified person to address this, but I'm going to find someone who can help." One of the worst-kept secrets in medicine is that doctors hate not knowing things. The best advice I got from a fellow physician was to simply treat the person in front of you. Treat their unique body, be open to their unique self. The more we welcome Queer, trans, and nonbinary people and people of color into the ranks of medicine, the more deeply and authentically this transformation will occur. Looking at the data on who is encouraged to apply for medical school, who gets in, and who receives sufficient support throughout the process to complete medical training, it's clear that we have a way to go.

Bradbury told me the story of a person who went for a first doctor's visit, which, as a Queer or nonbinary person, can be fraught. In the course of that first interaction, the doctor asked her patient what they wanted their genitals to be referred to as. And evidently that friend of hers broke down crying out of relief. The question telegraphed how respected and heard patients were in that office. Hearing that, I have increased my sensitivity to encourage patients to define their bodies for themselves. And that's not limited to genitalia; I want to be sensitive to your life history, too. Here are the ways I ask questions of my patients. If you're not wild about the way a doctor is speaking to you about these topics, feel free to respond using the phrasing below, or configure language for yourself and ask that the conversation be continued on your terms.

- **If you have sensitivity about your body parts and the way doctors speak about them, try telling your physician:** "I would like to share with you how I'd prefer that we talk about my genitals/body."
- **If your doctor asks about your sex and intimacy in a way that's noninclusive, respond by saying:** "That's actually not been my experience." You can describe your relationship as specifically as you feel comfortable with, and if the doctor requires more details for medical purposes, they will ask.
- **If your doctor says something that is triggering in terms of a history of disordered eating or eating disorder or doesn't address the topic but it's medically relevant, try saying:** "My relationship with food and eating has evolved over time and is medically relevant, so I'd like to share the triggers I have so they can be avoided."
- **If you have experienced medical trauma before—poor experiences with other doctors or care that felt coercive—you can say:** "In the past, I have had some not-so-great medical experiences that have stayed with me. I'd like to tell you about that." You can share the experience if you want, or you can just share what is triggering for you.

I wish I could say that I'm exemplary when it comes to terminology and sensitivity. I'm actively listening and learning and adjusting my practice accordingly. But I do flub it sometimes. My patients almost always correct me, which helps me provide better care for them and improve my communication with others. I am heartened to know that I create an environment in which they feel empowered and safe enough to engage in that dialogue. Interestingly, it comes easiest for younger patients. They have fewer hang-ups, either because they're young or because the society they're creating for themselves is less constraining than the one we were raised in. So I would say that the best approach to finding a medical partner on your menopause journey is not to look for the person who's the most up to date on their social justice vernacular; rather, find someone open to and interested in learning who invites you into a dialogue about your body and your mind. In a book that is all about celebrating the art of aging, let's also take a page from the youngsters, who are casting off labels and shame in a way that gives me hope for the future.

CHAPTER 8

Breaking Free from the Societal Bullshit

"I will be ungovernable."

Mona Eltahawy said those words, and I just about plotzed. Those words are an epiphany! They are fighting words. They are words of reclamation. If I were into tattoos, those words would stretch along my forearm. And Eltahawy is not talking out of school. Yes, it's a metaphor, but there was a time when a government truly sought to govern her.

She'd been a contributing opinion writer to the *New York Times* and the *Washington Post* for years; it had at one time been her dream job, but she had later realized that it had been constraining. It wasn't just that she couldn't swear (remember her love of cursing); her menopausal transformation was adding fuel to her activism and resistance in a way that those broadsheets couldn't handle. She stopped writing for the papers and began writing for subscribers to her Patreon account, where she could fully express all that she was feeling.

"Our bodies are doing exactly what they're meant to do," she said. "When we try to control those transitions, it's fascism of ourselves. I am transitioning out of the binary. Transitioning toward menopause. I am an anarchist. I will fight authoritarianism or power. I celebrate being postmenopausal. I have known all along this is who I am, and during menopause I was finally able to emerge toward that. The trauma and the pain is there because so much of this world is aimed at crushing us. Fascists, authoritarians, capitalists attempt to claim everything. Anarchists take back control power. I refuse to acknowledge the hierarchical power over me. This is a story of revolution."

There is scholarship behind her passion—lived experience, too, especially as an Egyptian woman who is an advocate for women oppressed by Middle Eastern regimes and religious traditions. Her voice was integral when, in 2011, the Arab Spring broke out and Egypt's president, Hosni Mubarak, was toppled from power. She appeared so often in the media that she was dubbed "the woman explaining Egypt to the West." And she was not on the sidelines; that November, she was beaten, sexually assaulted, and detained by Egyptian riot police and members of the Interior Ministry and military intelligence. For her, terms such as *fascism, authoritarianism,* and *anarchy* are not abstractions.

I have never gone through what Eltahawy has. At the same time, she's not been through what I have. We are both shaped by our lived experiences.

I will be ungovernable.

*   *   *

When I was buying my first house, the realtor explained what would be included in the sale. Imagine turning the house all the way over;

whatever stays attached belongs to the buyer, and whatever falls belongs to the seller. So the dishwasher, wall sconces, and ceiling fans would stay, but the backyard furniture and the rolling kitchen island with the Boos cutting board top would not.

I was reminded of that image when I was distinguishing between the emotional part of menopause, which is internal, and the physical part, which is external. If we were to turn ourselves over, the things that would stay attached—feelings of anxiety about the body we once understood and are struggling to relearn, sensations of menopause such as hot flashes and memory lapses that are an imposition, but also a greater appreciation of what our bodies are capable of—are personal to us and transcend time and place. A woman going through menopause in Delaware circa the 1960s could absolutely share these feelings with some future woman living in Oslo in 2044. What shakes to the bottom of the house is the extraneous stuff put on us by society—all that crap about feeling as though we have less worth because we are older and being desexualized on top of that. Our work is less valued for no reason besides ageism, never mind the fact that our experience in our chosen field makes us even more relevant. We are commended when we rail against gaining weight or going gray and chided when we don't. Things get way worse when you are a member of a community that capitalism, our government, our society, and even the medical system have actively undermined.

I've talked about the barriers that are erected around us as we age. I've named some but not all of them. But I don't want to dwell on them anymore. What I want to do is identify the world we want to live in and then chart a path from there.

Ask Denise Pines her destination, and here's what she says: "The ideal world is one where women aged fifty-plus are desired, valued, sought after, respected, and appreciated for her wisdom and contribution to her family and her community. I'd like us to be like the killer whale community, where the female is revered, has sex at eighty-five, and her male offspring follow her lead until they're twenty-five. When this happens, we'll never have these types of conversations again."

To be honest, I hadn't considered the killer whale community before Pines said that. A little reading revealed that among all the animals on the planet, only humans have a longer postreproductive life span. A study published in *Proceedings of the National Academy of Sciences of the United States of America* in 2019 explored the evolutionary purposes of postreproductive killer whales. Grandmothers are integral to helping their grandkids survive, which is essential to the overall survival of the species. The scientific literature actually calls this "the grandmother effect."

In humans, the grandmother effect is not so much to hunt for prey to feed the offspring, as it is in killer whales. Evolutionarily speaking, one prevailing take is that for humans in hunter-gather societies, having grandmothers around took some of the child-raising burden off mothers, which allowed them to have more kids. The presence of more offspring gives a species a greater chance of survival. And that holds true in modern times. Living with grandparents, or at least having them close by, can increase cognitive development in children, can help a family economically, can reduce loneliness, and can reduce stress—though researchers and anyone who's ever had in-laws stay with them for an extended amount of time acknowledge that it can nudge stress levels up, too.

The X factor in multigenerational households is social connection. Like killer whales, we are social creatures. Here are some of the benefits of social connection: a higher-functioning immune system, better mood regulation and lower rates of depression, greater self-esteem, and a longer life span. I'll add another thing to the list, as it relates to the social BS that we are burdened with as we age: social connections create a barrier of protection to fend off assaults on our self-worth. It underpins Elderqueer and the Menopause Bootcamp. Making those connections and feeling safe enough to share what's going on inside us is a powerful way to release our burdens. Being there for someone and responding to them with what they need—empathy, problem solving, affirmation, even disagreement—can help them overcome their obstacles and also help *you* create patterns of thought that will help you respond to obstacles in your own path. And just being with people you care for makes life more fun.

I heard a covid story from a woman named Charlene, who lives in a suburb of Chicago. The majority of the residents of her apartment building are older women, many of whom are either widows or have never been married. Worried about the loneliness and isolation caused by the pandemic, a group of residents banded together to make some capital improvements. Into an unused section of the parking garage, they dragged benches and outdoor chairs, placing them in a socially distant circle with a big table in the middle. Every Wednesday in the early evening, they met there for dinner, with each member of the group taking a turn ordering food from a local restaurant. They would be down there for hours, laughing and talking, sharing their anxieties and coping techniques, talking about their families and their dating lives. "The dinner group was great," she said, "but every Sunday we discussed a movie, keeping everyone challenged intellectually and verbally." If a person didn't show up to one of the meetups, the next day, they'd open their door to find notes from their neighbors checking in to make sure they were okay or a plate of cookies or fruit bars to help cheer them up if they were feeling down. Though the pandemic's impacts on us have been awful (as I wrote this, the emergency department I work in was groaning under the burden the Delta variant had placed on it), Charlene spoke about the meetups as an invigorating surprise that would have never happened in normal times.

To me, that has been one of the lessons of the covid pandemic: it brought into stark focus what we truly need. And human connection is at the top of the list. Even as this pandemic hopefully recedes soon, let's no longer take for granted the meaningfulness of connection with people; real, in-person connection. Here's a fun little study from 2014 that drives home the point. Each day for two weeks, scientists surveyed 404 healthy adults about the amount of interpersonal conflict they had in their lives and the number of hugs they received. Then the participants were exposed to the virus that causes the common cold. People who felt that they had social support as well as hugs were less likely to get sick, and when they did, they had less severe symptoms. The findings suggest that receiving a hug from a trusted person made the recipient of the embrace feel supported, and the more hugging you get, the greater the stress reduction. We do know that physical contact is good for people; it releases the feel-good hormone oxytocin, for example. One or the other, or a combination of both, seemed to give the immune systems of the study subjects a boost to fend off infection. (To be clear: hugs do *not* fend off covid-19.)

In the last part, I'll help you prepare for your best no-hang-ups transition and postmenopause life. But the best recommendation I can give you is to stoke the social connections around you. Gather your friends who are also in the menopause transition, share with them some of the medical information you have learned in this book about how to cope with the impacts of it on their bodies and lives, and then encourage them to share what their experiences have been like. Share your favorite methods of cooling off during a hot flash, the best brand of sweat-wicking pajamas, and the name of the gynecologist who really listened to what you were going through. And talk about all the other stuff: how parenting is going or how your relationship is evolving. Help a friend gussy up her profile on a dating app or her résumé. Plan a group hiking trip or even a walk around a local park. Be supportive, and accept support. Be vulnerable and openhearted when people are vulnerable with you. Listen and be in the moment. Reflect on your experiences. Do you have people in your life you can be vulnerable with? The problems that pin us down the hardest, that shove us into the shade of shame, so often lighten when we share what's on our minds.

The other antidote to loneliness is gratitude, being appreciative for what you have. I like this definition: "Gratitude is a positive, socially oriented emotion that plays an impressive role in building and maintaining social relationships and increasing intrapersonal well-being, including improving physical health and decreasing loneliness. Further, gratitude can be cultivated. Research has shown that the simple 'three good things' exercise increases feelings of gratitude with concomitant [associated] boosts in positive outcomes." So wrote psychology researchers at Gonzaga University in 2019 in a paper documenting gratitude's capacity to treat loneliness in older adults. The "three good things" exercise they reference involves writing down three things you're grateful for. When we do that and meditate on it, we inevitably appreciate our interconnectedness: with our friends, family, colleagues, mentors, even strangers with whom we have a short interaction. Some people go beyond expressing gratitude for others, giving thanks to nature, medical or technological advancements, even a higher power.

The researchers at Gonzaga were particularly interested in loneliness among adults sixty-five and older because it's so common in that age group and can have deleterious health effects (the inverse also holds true; feeling connected improves health). They did a study in which two groups of people were asked to fill out questionnaires related to gratitude, subjective well-being, loneliness, health, daily activities, and general positivity. Half of the participants were also asked to do a gratitude exercise every day. They found that those in the gratitude group felt lower levels of loneliness and reported better health. On the days that they were feeling the highest levels of gratitude, they felt even better and had fewer health symptoms, such as poor appetite and chest pain.

The researchers also found that the amount of gratitude an individual feels changes from day to day and predicts how they feel healthwise, as well as how lonely they are. That makes sense to me. If you've ever gone through a big medical experience—cancer, diagnosis of a chronic disease, a cardiac event—you will have experienced the roller coaster of healing. Some days feel positive, and some feel positively terrible. A friend told me that for her, some chemo treatments felt as though they were a gift given by angels (nurses) to help her body evolve past the illness. Others felt as though poison were being pumped into her wrecked veins by strangers in an eight-hour torture session. You can probably imagine where her gratitude was on each of those days. By the way, her friends were there regardless. She reflected that it wasn't a failure of their social connection that some days were "healing" and other days were "torture." Because if it hadn't been for the love from the nurses and her friends, instead of having good treatments and bad treatments, she would've had bad treatments and abysmal treatments.

If you haven't done so already, start cultivating gratitude. Some people write down a few things they're grateful for in the morning and use them to guide their day. Others are evening gratitude people, writing their reflections and finding peace as they go to bed for their nightly reset. Find gratitude for your body. We are so quick to pick her apart. Give her some appreciation. And she's about to save you so much money on pads and tampons, so let her know that you appreciate her. It truly makes everything about menopause better.

PART IV

Onward, Together

Your No-Hang-ups,
Live-Your-Best-Life,
Menopause Transition
and Beyond Plan

"Filling the cup." Second to the analogy of the caterpillar morphing from the chrysalis (goo) phase into a butterfly, "filling the cup" is the comparison I hear the most when I speak with people about menopause. Which activities in your day-to-day life fill your cup, and which empty it? Who fills your cup, and who asks that you fill theirs? When you think about self-esteem and your sense of self-worth, does the exercise drain or fill your cup? Which emotions give you more energy, and which sap it?

The metaphor works well enough. But I'm not crazy about things that are mutually exclusive or strictly binary. Here's an example: A friend has an emergency and needs to go out of town for a night, maybe two. Can he drop the kids with you and your partner? It goes without saying that watching two kids is a huge inconvenience and requires you to drop everything, take a day off work, and take out a streaming subscription to Disney+. It throws a wrench into things: meetings have to be rescheduled, errands pushed back. But you fall over yourself to do it. Why? Well, for one, you want to be a good friend. Also, the kids' father has been there for you through tough times, and you're gratified at the opportunity to return the favor, even though it hints at a crisis. And if you're being honest, eating pizza and watching *The Mandalorian* doesn't sound so bad.

The question is: Does doing this fill your cup, or does it empty it?

We women are often told that we're the perpetual givers. That we run around making sure everyone else is fine without engaging in self-care. And along with that, we're asked who fills our cup? That's something Mary Thompson, my Ayurveda mentor, said. I agree. I've experienced it myself. The distribution of labor in the United States assigns household tasks and childrearing to women. The pandemic made it worse, driving women out of the workforce and setting us—

and particularly people of color—back years or decades in terms of promotions and earning potential.

Here's what I'm suggesting with the made-up SOS example. The same activity can empty and fill your cup at the same time. Parenting is incredibly cup draining and miraculously cup filling at the same time. Being a doctor feels similar (though to be honest, treating patients and my relationship with them is cup filling, and all of the administrative bullshit dumps out the cup). Is exercise "filling" or "emptying"? For me, it's both. Now, if you are in a bad relationship or a thankless job or you just can't live under the yoke of the patriarchal, capitalistic, binary sex and gender system one minute longer and your cup is dry as the Atacama Desert, by all means, *blow that shit up*. (Mona Eltahawy taught me that.)

* * *

The *aha!* moments of the menopausal transition come fast and furiously. There's no one else in the world who knows our bodies better than ourselves, so understand your body and advocate for yourself; you're the only person who's going to put your needs first, so treat yourself with kindness; if you're lucky, a third to a half of your life will be spent postmenopause, so make those years count. If you were looking for things to become suddenly clear and simple, that won't happen. We will never be in a position to do only those things that fill us up and none of those that drag us down.

So I'd like to propose a different paradigm, one that will be the heart of your No-Hang-ups, Live-Your-Best-Life, Menopause Transition and Beyond Plan. Keep track of input and output *in all the parts of your life*. If you're nearing the end of a yearlong work project and you're in a race to the finish, you're going to be expending physical and mental energy at a higher clip than usual. The output gauge is speeding like a Formula 1 race car. You need to meet that with increased input. Can you sleep in over the weekend? (It's not a long-term solution to chronic sleep deficit, but it can feel good once in a while.) Ask your family to do more household chores to lighten your load at home, giving you a few more minutes for meditation or body movement. I'm not suggesting that skipping doing the dishes in exchange for chanting "Om" will give you extra pep in your step. What it can do is create a little more focus, a hair more patience, an extra ounce of creativity.

Conversely, sometimes we find ourselves brimming with input. Or our input-output level changes dramatically owing to a life change. Consider what happens when your kids leave the house or you switch to a less demanding job. The activities that you have always allotted energy to are suddenly reduced. You miss the entryway full of scattered shoes, the Monday-through-Friday morning routine. If you are feeling depressed or as though your energy is sapped, sometimes the paradoxical fix is *increasing* your output. Engaging in new, challenging hobbies is output. Doing service for others is output. Trying new forms of body movement is output.

The important thing is to see your life in all its dimensions. Move the input-output levers in ways that make you feel good and also connect you with the people and places around you. I hesitate to say that you should try to "find balance." It's trite and for some people unattainable. It doesn't even mean anything! Even a teeter-totter achieves only momentary balance. It's about moments of clarity, room to breathe and expand. When that happens, if you're feeling yanked around by life, your supposed failure at finding balance makes you feel bad on top of already feeling bad. That's a habit you've got to break *now*. Do Not Feel Bad About Something and Then Feel Bad About Feeling Bad. There is absolutely no sense in feeling bad twice. It's another form of self-punishment. If I had a penny for every patient who missed one, three, twelve years of exams with me and sheepishly apologized for it . . . My response: "What? Why? You're here now!" That is what matters, truly and only. I won't participate in your self-flagellation, and I will gently poke holes in that kind of thinking while making you laugh—while you're wearing a paper gown. It's a special moment.

I find imagery helpful. Imagine yourself peering around the inputs and outputs of your life, in control of how your energy flows. You are a pilot in a cockpit, looking at all of the dials and gauges, making adjustments that respond to where you are in your flight. You are an orchestra conductor, listening to the players tune their instruments, calling on each section as it fits into the symphony: brass, woodwind, strings, percussion. You are Padma Lakshmi, cooking a fabulous meal, adding ingredients and spices, turning the heat up and down, knowing what pot needs your attention and what can simmer, tasting as you go.

* * *

It should go without saying that no one plan will work for everyone. I want to make some overall suggestions and options that work for a lot of people. A question I'm always asked is "How will I know if it's working?" Let's first dissect what "working" means. For me, it comes down to two things: creating consistency and peace.

Consistency

The healthiest way to live is to adopt a lifestyle that you're able to sustain. Deciding that you're going to do high-intensity exercise at 6:00 a.m., intermittently fast and not eat until 2:00 p.m., and take a battery of thirty different supplements at the perfect intervals during the day is not sustainable. Here's what's sustainable for me. Ideally, I do weight training and boxing twice a week with my trainer, yoga once a week, and gyrotonics—it's like Pilates on acid and rotational—once a week. I walk at least three miles twice a week, including to and from the office (in—*gasp!*—Los Angeles) and to the hospital on weekends when I am on call. And I garden. Thanks to our balmy SoCal climate, I am out in my veggie garden, either planting, tending, pruning, or watering, oftentimes alongside my partner, almost every day.

After a childhood of beachcombing and the love of the California coast that is my home, I will be spending more time in the Mojave Desert this year. I love being outdoors in the peace and quiet, but my busy schedule doesn't always allow me to take part in a grand adventure, so starting during the pandemic, I began to drink homemade ginger-turmeric tea with Irish sea moss, lime, apple cider vinegar, and honey, along with a cup of coffee, outside on my front porch or in my backyard in the morning as often as I can. I go barefoot most of the time I'm at home and have had to train myself to wear the Crocs I inherited from my mom in the garden since I have stepped on more than one bee.

I eat breakfast if I'm hungry—usually only after a big workout— and occasionally go out to brunch on weekends. I try to take my own lunch to work on weekdays, because as easy and delish as food ordered in can be, it is a wild card of sugar and salt, plus I always eat more than I meant to and feel gross later on. I have a grapefruit for a snack almost every afternoon, and we really don't like to eat past about 7:30 p.m. I try to remember to breathe and give thanks for the food I eat before I gorge—even when taking lunch at my desk while I answer calls and emails most days. We are in bed chillaxing and rarely up later than 9:30 p.m. on a "school night." I love a good chocolate dessert or ice cream, but my partner has a weird thing about making sure the surface of the ice cream is even when we are done eating directly from the carton. I invent cocktails with herbs and spicy peppers from our garden. Researching and writing this book has had a profound influence on my attitude toward eating, satiety, craving, and gentleness with my softening body.

I love the quiet solitude of an early morning, and if I don't have to be in the operating room early, I get up at 6:00 a.m. and spend two to three hours on morning routines, meal prep, exercise, and meditation before heading to work or hospital rounds before clinic hours. Sleep is a long-term issue; I was a napper from way back, and it helped me as a young resident and mom. But due to the demands of my profession, I am a very light sleeper. I never had trouble falling asleep when I was younger; that is not always the case now. I try to get seven to eight hours of shut-eye a night but often fail to do so.

To be clear: what I just described is imperfect. It is overly influenced by my work. My career right now is going through a period of transformation. Like many doctors at this point in my career, I'm looking for ways to take my decades of experience and lessons learned and share them with more people. That's how the Menopause Bootcamp came into being. But any ob-gyn who is involved in labor and delivery knows that her schedule is not hers to dictate. In order to eke out something that looks like consistency, I focus on my inputs. For me, the most important one has always been body movement. A fitness nut since college graduation, I've found that when I am able to lift weights and get my heart rate up, I feel a million times better. My mood improves. My body does what it needs to do (being a doctor can be incredibly physically demanding). And I have the endurance to continue.

Many of us have little practice in developing consistency. Anyone who has ever dieted to lose weight—and my guess is that this includes a lot of us—has most likely done so inconsistently. If you've ever gone gung ho into a diet that started with a bang and ended with a whimper—called yo-yo dieting—you have proven to yourself that extremes are too hard to maintain. So start with a couple small changes, and I'm talking really small. (This is a method adapted from the writing of B. J. Fogg, PhD, a behavioral scientist at Stanford University.) Meditate for ninety seconds before you hop into the shower. Write three sentences in your gratitude journal before you go to bed. Spend ten minutes before dinner doing something in nature, such as walking on the grass without your shoes on or sitting on a bench and looking at water. Do these every day for a month. You're not limited to a minute and a half of meditation or writing just a few lines. But those are the minimums. If you do that consistently for thirty days, then increase the goals a little: meditate for three minutes; write a paragraph; take a walk outside after dinner.

Why does this approach work? It creates little wins every day, and the feeling of accomplishment it creates reinforces the habit and creates momentum. It helps you learn whether a habit is right for you. If ninety seconds of meditation is too much, maybe that's not the behavior to cultivate *right now*. It doesn't mean that you will never be a meditator! But something's not working at the moment, and it's better to let it go and try a different behavior. This helps create a foundation to accomplish bigger goals to which you want to devote more attention, focus, and consistency—things such as starting a new business, getting back into swimming, or volunteering in your free time.

I want to be clear: I am not suggesting that you need to fill up your life. You don't need to gorge yourself on kale, open an Etsy shop, or train to hike the Pacific Crest Trail. In fact, you should do the opposite. Again, I'll point you to the work of the Nap Ministry, which sees rest as a form of social justice. What consistency can build is a body and mind that feels good to you, enabling you to engage in the world in a way that is spiritually fulfilling. That takes us to the next goal.

Peace

The life I try to cultivate is one in which I am at peace: with my body, my work decisions, my close relationships, and my impact on the world around me, including the environment. One of the hardest things to achieve has been bodily peace, particularly during the menopause transition. As we've discussed, the feeling a lot of us have is that our body has morphed into one we don't understand. The disconnect between body and mind is conflict—the opposite of peace. I am begrudgingly accepting the weight gain that has come with menopause, but I am still in conflict with it (hence "begrudgingly"—I'm working on it, and more on that later). I am not at peace with my new body, but peace is what I am striving for. The end goal doesn't have to be that you love every inch of your body every single day but rather that you are at peace with your body and in that peace find purpose: the peace of work decisions, of staying with a job, moving companies, pivoting into a new industry, or retiring. Conflict in relationships is a smog that hangs over everything; creating peace in relationships is like burning sage over the other parts of your life. I want also to highlight being at peace with our environment. We can no longer ignore the fact of global warming; that animals are tortured in the process of factory farming; and that this country has been corporatized, leading to an all-out assault on both the natural world and those people who are most vulnerable. That one sentence is almost too much to bear. I am looking for a pathway to peace in all of that. My struggle is singular and small, but I would feel much better knowing that you are in this struggle with me. All of us together—we have found our people.

All of the actions of our day, in all of its many varieties—ninety seconds of meditation, a few minutes of oil treatment in the shower, three hours doing a gynecological surgery, half an hour on the phone with my brother, forty-five minutes of veggie burgers and fries with friends, an hour of intimacy with my partner—the goal is for the sum of that to give you peace. Lord knows that peace is hard to achieve when we live in a country where the police gun down people of color, where there are domestic terrorist assaults on the Capitol, where the right to an abortion is under attack, where some schools are falling apart while others look like cathedrals, and where the rights of nonbinary and trans people are denied. However, we can't let injustice crush us. That's how those who are in power want us to feel: powerless, railroaded, submissive.

Now it's time to connect the dots. Self-care, performed consistently every day via what we consume and how we spend our time, move our bodies, and connect with people, are all input. (Ayurveda in action!) Increasing our input means that we have more energy to expend and can create more output. We can give more to our friends and family and causes that are important to us. We can use behavioral changes to push society toward justice and protect the environment. We can stand more firmly in our convictions, knowing that our doing so might piss some people off, but that's okay. We might experience discomfort or have to make sacrifices. Those things won't break you when you're topping off your tank. You can't be an agent of change on an empty tank. Power up in healthy ways, and expend your power in meaningful ways. After all, menopause is a time of *action*—a time to expand and expend our accumulated wisdom. We are the killer whale grandmothers. The entire species needs us in order to survive! This, for me, is an avenue to achieving peace.

CHAPTER 9

Eat for Health and Joy

In Ayurveda, the two hubs of the body are the brain, or the "mind," and the gut. That knowledge provides a guide for eating. What works for you, your particular needs, and the ethical decisions you make about your food consumption are so highly personal that I don't think it's responsible to give orders about what is healthy for you to eat, what specific diet is right for you. My goal throughout this book when it comes to food choices is to give you some information about what we know about the effects of certain foods on the body and offer some ideas to boost consistency and peace. Inherent to that is this advice: if any book a doctor hands you has a list of "good" foods and "bad" foods, feel free to drop it in the bin. In general, excess is unhealthy; consuming tons of sugar is not great, but neither is consuming a ton of raw celery. But the first one won't kill you, and the second won't save you (nor will it bring you peace). The same goes for the idea of a continuous glucose monitor unless it's prescribed by a doctor to track diabetes. Those are some of the tools of orthorexia—a type of disordered eating that manifests itself as an obsession with healthy eating. Based on my experience as a physician and after talking to experts in nutrition, I want to share a few general guidelines.

Eat Mostly Plants

You've heard this from me before: try to limit the amount of animal products you consume. I aim for 80 percent plant based. There's some research suggesting that animal proteins can be hard for the body to process, and as we age, the efficiency of our digestive system naturally decreases, as do the levels of our digestive enzymes. Eastern medicine teaches us that cooked vegetables are easier on our system; if you've been loading up on salads and vegetable smoothies lately and you are feeling bloated or gassy, it may be that your body is struggling to break down the raw roughage. Cooking your vegetables should improve the situation. And a note about packaged food: it's often marketed as being healthy because it is plant based or gluten free or uses only ancient grains. I would avoid conflating the two. This doesn't mean you need to avoid packaged food altogether. But to the extent that you can do so, eating whole foods is preferable. The way that I think about it, from a medical standpoint, is this: your body was designed to eat lots of different kinds of foods. The historical record suggests that we are certainly made to eat plants, and some people argue that beginning to eat meat was an important part of evolution. Our digestive tract knows what to do with all of these things: grains and vegetables, fruits and sugarcane, olives and legumes. But when foods are processed—when they contain lab-made ingredients or are manipulated—our body isn't as good at utilizing their nutrition. It may store macronutrients instead of processing them. I'm not saying that packaged foods are bad or evil. They're not. They're just food that comes from packages. But if you are a person who tends to get a high percentage of your calories from packaged foods, you might think about lowering that percentage to see how your energy, feeling of satiety, and mood respond.

Eat Locally and Seasonally, with Variety

This is another tenet of Ayurveda. The body is connected with the earth; eating food that is grown near us means that it's fresher, and eating seasonally helps us connect with the life cycle of nature. It's no coincidence that juicy berries and hydrating watermelons are available in the summertime, and hearty gourds and cruciferous vegetables pop in the fall. There's a piece of advice that has some nice imagery: "Eat the rainbow." The color of produce can be an indicator of its nutritional profile. By eating a variety of fruits and vegetables, you're getting a diverse set of nutrients. And please don't exclude any one food or macronutrient from your diet. If you read advice that carbohydrates are bad or that they spike your blood sugar, please know that your body *needs* carbohydrates. They're the body's preferred energy source, particularly for the brain. If your doctor has instructed you to be mindful of your blood sugar level—it's true that diabetes can emerge during and after the menopausal transition—eat carbs at the same time as protein.

Avoid Fad Diets

These include the seemingly scientific-backed ones such as intermittent fasting (IF), which calls for eating for a few hours each day and fasting for the rest, and carb cycling, in which you eat zero carbs on some days and some carbs on other days. Though there are some interesting data behind some of these diets, the results of all of them are mixed at best. For instance, the pro-IF people say that your body's metabolism has a circadian rhythm and you should eat in sync with that. But it seems that the weight loss some people enjoy while following IF is simply due to calorie restriction. More than anything else, few of these studies have involved women, and hardly any have included postmenopausal women. Again, this defect in study design goes back to the belief that the menstrual cycle is confounding and impossible to control for, what with all the changing hormones. But in reality, the metabolism of people with uteruses differs in order to facilitate pregnancy. If your partner has tried IF and he's lost weight in a snap, and you've tried it and either it hasn't worked or you've been left feeling hangry and lethargic, proponents of these diets would say that something is wrong with *you*. It's not. The problems lie with the diet.

Listen to Your Body; It Will Tell You What It Needs

This is aligned with intuitive eating, a practice in which you respond to your body's cues of hunger, fullness, and cravings. We shouldn't need to think about intuitive eating; left alone, our bodies are really good at regulating what they need. But modern society has screwed us up, particularly the diet culture that's been pervasive for the last eighty years or so. If you experience a craving, it's totally fine to respond to that craving. I have a friend who is a pescatarian who has gone through three surgeries in the past two years. During the two weeks after each surgery, she has craved animal protein. She does not eat meat for ethical reasons, so you can imagine her distress over this. She surmises, however, that her body wants it as part of the healing process. So postoperatively, she pulls a Phoebe from the show *Friends*, and her dad, a devoted carnivore, goes vegetarian for several meals to make everything right with the universe. On that note . . .

Be Flexible

Being reasonably flexible helps to develop consistency. Inflexibility caused by restriction can lead to binge eating behaviors, which can spur restrictions, and you see where this is going. Of course, diagnosed food allergies, GI or autoimmune disorders, being on certain medications or treatments, and other medical conditions can reduce the amount of flexibility that you have.

Be on the Lookout for Disordered Eating

It's something I hear over and over: during menopause, eating disorders or disordered eating patterns that people thought they had left in the past reemerge. The body changes they go through during the transition can trigger simmering, unresolved, or hibernating eating disorders. I have personally experienced anxiety over the physical changes I have been seeing in the mirror and feeling whenever I step into a pair of jeans. So I phoned my friend Robyn L. Goldberg, RDN, CED-RD-S, a registered dietitian nutritionist and the author of *The Eating Disorder Trap: A Guide for Clinicians and Loved Ones*, and she offered some incredible insights.

"Women have the physical shape we have because it's what's required from a survival standpoint," she said. When we're born, our body shape and composition are pretty well baked into our genes. Studies have shown that twins separated at birth grow up to have similar body composition, meaning that our genetics play a bigger role in the bodies we inhabit than our childhood environment does. And people who menstruate have body patterns that seem to exist to facilitate fertility and pregnancy. According to Goldberg, before puberty, a girl has about 12 percent body fat; once we enter puberty, our hard wiring bumps that to 17 percent to enable safe ovulation and menstruation.

Mature women have around 22 percent body fat, which is what is needed to maintain and survive a full-term, healthy pregnancy.

When fertility declines during the menopausal transition, so does metabolism—by around 15 percent, Goldberg said. "The average woman, during menopause, adds twelve to fifteen pounds, usually settling in the waist," she said. "Yes, clothes feel snugger, but the estrogen that is stored in fat cells is necessary to help preserve our bone loss. The lower metabolism rate helps to keep this fat in place."

As I've mentioned, weight gain is probably the number one complaint I hear from my patients, and all they want to hear is how they can get it off. In the past, I've recommended (and tried for myself) diet plans such as WW (formerly Weight Watchers), Noom, Nutrisystem, Atkins, Whole30, and others. For a time, I thought that the accountability and community, all within a science-backed process that some of these claim, were great. But I came to realize what others have: when people "succeed" on these diets—when they lose weight—they credit the program. However, if the program doesn't lead to the desired weight loss, they blame themselves. It's the logic that springs out of these diets' advertising: "It works for *everybody*, and it's *so easy to follow!*" Our bodies want to maintain homeostasis. They don't like big changes in weight, so no wonder weight loss can be so difficult and hard to maintain.

After the research I've done, and after speaking with many respected experts in the field, I now eschew dieting for weight loss. I know that some physicians will eschew *me* for that. But studies that find causality between living in a bigger body and diseases such as cancer and heart disease are unreliable (if you want to deep dive into this, the work of Lindo Bacon, PhD, the author of the book *Health at Every Size: The Surprising Truth About Your Weight*, is a great starting point).

I have patients who had seemingly moved past dieting as well—that is, until they reached the menopausal transition. The changes in their body, particularly weight gain, were a trigger for them. I have never experienced an eating disorder, though there have been periods in my life when I've felt body dysmorphia, a condition in which a person becomes fixated on what they perceive to be the negative parts of their bodies.

Meg Bradbury, a certified antidiet nutritionist and the founder of Elderqueer, spoke about this. She's dealt with disordered eating in the past. For her, part of the menopause transition was "making sure my recovery process was still intact. There's so much diet culture, diet rhetoric, 'gooporexia'"—referring to Gwyneth Paltrow's brand Goop, with its sometimes extreme or out-of-reach views on health and nutrition. "My disorder is always there, but I have the tools to deal with the behaviors," she says. Still, the menopause onslaught can be real. Bradbury recalled, "My energy is shit, I'm feeling like shit; these feelings compromised my recovery process." Couple that with the messaging from your doctor to make sure to keep weight gain at bay plus all the ads hawking a magic supplement to lose your body fat. "It made me question my own sanity," she said.

From Bradbury's work in Elderqueer, together with her working and personal relationships up to its establishment, she said that in the Queer community, you'll find folks who are in recovery and who understand body shame. One way to find peace, she told me, is to release the idea that menopause's natural weight gain is "letting our bodies go," as opposed to "letting our bodies be." Bradbury is one of the many people I talked with who brought up the fact that menopause is pathologized, seen as something to fix, combat, hide, and be ashamed of. It's the menopause stigma. It's foolish not to recognize that fear of gaining weight is part and parcel of that. We have hidden behind the flimsy excuse that we accept all parts of menopause except for weight gain, as we have to keep our weight down in order to maintain good health. If keeping off eight or ten or twenty pounds means that you have to subsist on 1,300 calories a day and follow a regimented diet, you are constantly miserable because you are hungry and depriving yourself, you exercise hard every day of the week and are constantly obsessed with the scale or your clothing size, that's no way to live. You might not be getting the nutrition you need, especially at this time, when your body is going through an important transformation and requires energy. Working out hard without truly replenishing yourself adds further stress to your already stressed system. If you need another reason to walk away from diet culture: it's not empowering. We are not taking care of ourselves; we are conforming to a societal body ideal, to our collective detriment. This sounds harsh, I know. But I'm trying to say it plainly because it goes head-to-head with so much mainstream messaging: beautiful people—which if you're a woman means you're thin and if you're a man means you're thin and muscular—have carte blanche to live a full life, while the rest of us have to go do crunches in a corner. I'm done with it. If you want to start dating but are waiting until you lose some weight, just go out and date. Do you really want to go to the French Riviera, but you don't like your pants size? Book the damn trip. And while you're beating yourself up for eating ice cream with your friends, you're undermining that happy time with your friends. Life does not stop while you're stalking your bathroom scale.

If you have a healthy lifelong relationship with food and your body, that is totally awesome. If you have struggled with an eating disorder or disordered eating in the past and you've learned to move beyond it, that is totally awesome. If it's something you still battle or it's arisen during the menopausal transition, I completely feel for you, and it doesn't have to be like this forever. If you're not sure whether the relationship you have with food and eating is a healthy one, one prompt Goldberg uses with her clients is to reflect on how many hours of the day they think about eating or not eating. Every hour? Multiple times per hour? Is that comfortable for you? "It's a problem if it's consuming every waking moment," she said.

Have you ever engaged in "body checking"? It's the impulse to take constant assessments of your body: weighing yourself numerous times a day; touching, poking, or grabbing parts of your body that you don't like; obsessively standing in front of a mirror, taking an inventory of the things you want to change. This can be another indicator that your relationship with your body could use some professional attention.

If you are experiencing an untreated or reemerging eating disorder, I suggest that you find a therapist, specially trained registered dietitian, or group help, including group therapy and Overeaters Anonymous. If you're like me and want to tamp down on negative thoughts that you're having about your eating and/or your body, Goldberg shared some ideas. The first is to start identifying the unhealthy voice that crops up regarding food. There's an automatic voice and a healthy voice. For instance, if you have a craving for a bagel, the automatic thought might be "I'm fat, so I can't eat a bagel." The alternate, healthy thought is more logical. It possesses no judgment or negativity around food. "Bagels are delicious. I'm going to enjoy it. One bagel isn't a deal breaker. I'm not bingeing on a lot of bagels."

I also really like these mantras that she devised to combat the negative self-talk about food:

◆ "I am worthy and deserving to eat delicious food."
◆ "I am worthy to honor my cravings."
◆ "All bodies require some carbohydrates, some protein, some fat."
◆ "If I am constantly computing, am I able to taste and savor the deliciousness around me?"

Finally, take a look at your relationships. I've talked about how powerful the people in your life are and how a group of like-minded people going through the same experience can be a force for good in one another's lives. There is another side to that coin: friends and family can spur unhealthy behaviors, too. Groups of women in particular who are feeling insecure about their bodies or eating can look around for validation, instigating a conversation that props up disordered eating behaviors and body dysmorphia rather than extinguishing them. You've probably experienced a version of that. You're at a restaurant, and one person is hemming and hawing over the salad ("I should really get one!") and, say, the pasta ("It sounds so delicious, but I really shouldn't."). The kind response from friends is often something like "Oh, go for the pasta. Treat yourself!" That makes a value judgment on each of the dishes: salad = good, pasta = bad. *Food is not good or bad, good or evil.* Here are a few strategies to develop healthier conversations about bodies and food with your friends.

- At a restaurant, don't ask the group about their food choices, and don't offer yours if you are asked. Everyone should be free to decide what they want to eat, without input from others. If your tablemates begin chatting about what dish they're opting for in an unhealthy way, try to redirect the conversation or interject something such as "I think they both sound delicious. What are you craving? I would choose that."
- If people start engaging in body talk, either about themselves or others, try being honest. "Could we change topics? I don't really like talking about weight and dieting." Or "I'm trying to establish a better relationship with my eating and my body, and I'm feeling triggered by this conversation. Let's talk about something else. Have you checked out the TV show *Better Things* yet? Pamela Adlon is *incredible!*"
- If you aren't able to get through a meal with a certain group of friends or family without the conversation turning to body judgment, it might be time to decline dinner invites with those people. Do something else! Organize an outing to a driving range, attend a sporting event, pool some money and go on a shopping spree with a list of items needed by a local homeless shelter. Find ways to engage with one another without making it about food.

This kind of change takes practice, because it requires undoing a ton of societal—and internalized—pressure. In the case of our idealism of skinniness, research now lays out a convincing argument that its origins derive from racism. Sabrina Strings, PhD, associate professor of sociology at the University of California, Irvine, and the author of the book *Fearing the Black Body: The Racial Origins of Fat Phobia*, discovered that women's dying to be thin dates back at least as far as the nineteenth century. "[Magazines such as *Harper's Bazaar*] were unapologetic in stating that [thinness] was the proper form for Anglo-Saxon Protestant women," Strings told NPR. "And so it was important that women ate as little as was necessary in order to show their Christian nature and also their racial superiority."

For those who have experienced body dysmorphia, disordered eating, eating disorders, orthorexia, and other complicated relationships with their bodies and food, the origins are diverse. They can be mixed up with one's parents or an ex or current partner, have a cultural basis, be linked with one's work, have their origin in social pressure starting at school—they're personal to each person. Sometimes it's not just the food part that needs addressing, but the causative relationship or the mark it left on you. This can be a daunting undertaking if you've only begun dealing with it or if you dealt with it years ago and thought you'd put it behind you. But the goal is pretty much the same: to be at peace—with your body and what you put into it. The reward for that is opening your life up to more pleasure. If your mind's not trolling your food decisions, always thinking about your body, it has more time to spend on living in the present and responding to your needs and the needs of those around you. And it opens up the opportunity for more pleasure.

Eat for Your GI Tract's Health

One of the most exciting advancements in medical understanding in the last decade or so has been a fuller understanding of the body's microbiomes: skin, mouth, vagina, and gastrointestinal tract. A microbiome is a conglomeration of billions of organisms—bacteria, fungi, protozoa, yeast, and viruses—that live in various parts of our bodies. In fact, the human cellular population is 90 percent these things and 10 percent us! Kind of weird to think about, right? Some of them act symbiotically, meaning that they help us and we help them. Sometimes the balance within a microbiome gets thrown off, which can make us feel not great or even sick. A yeast infection is one such example. However, the importance of the gut microbiome, in particular, is something Ayurvedic practitioners have emphasized for centuries—they just don't use the same language as Western doctors and scientists.

I found a kindred spirit in Emeran Mayer, MD, a distinguished research professor in the Departments of Medicine, Physiology, Psychiatry and Biobehavioral Sciences at the David Geffen School of Medicine at UCLA, who studies, among other things, the linkages between the brain and the gut microbiomes and is the author of *The Mind-Gut Connection: How the Hidden Conversation Within Our Bodies Impacts Our Mood, Our Choices, and Our Overall Health* and *The Gut-Immune Connection: How Understanding the Connection Between Food and Immunity Can Help Us Regain Our Health*. He told me that twenty years ago, he helped organize a multidisciplinary symposium on this topic. "Forty percent of the people we invited were top neuroscientists, and the other sixty percent were nontraditional healers, including Ayurvedic practitioners, Tibetan monks, and Native American healers," he told me. For four days, the attendees started the day at 6:00 a.m. with meditations, and they stayed up until 2:00 a.m., participating in impromptu workshops, comparing notes on neurology, gastroenterology, and ancient healing systems. They were exploring the body's interconnectedness; it sounds pretty obvious that each of the body's systems should influence the others, but Western medicine has a tendency to silo the GI tract from the brain, the pulmonary system, and so on.

Mayer's research has gone on to show that the body is a big network of systems, and the gut is a hub. In fact, it's *the* hub. The gut has the most connections to the other systems of the body. "No other organs have these dense connections and interconnectedness," he said. And so the health of the GI tract impacts the hormonal system, nervous system, immune system, and more. He and others are learning how the composition and functionality of the gut microbiome can influence things such as the development of Alzheimer's disease and breast cancer, mental health and depression, and the immune system and overall health. The gut microbiome may be a key factor in how well you heal after a big medical event, too.

There's even something called the *estrobolome*, "those bacteria that have the genetic capability to metabolize estrogen," wrote researchers at the Breast Cancer Survivorship Institute at Kaiser Permanente in Sacramento. "Results of recent investigations have suggested that specific hormones, particularly estrogen, and the gut microbiome might act synergistically in the development of obesity, type 2 diabetes mellitus (T2DM), and cancer." We're still learning more about the composition of the microbiota and the effect that the presence or absence of certain bacteria has. Nevertheless, there are ways in which you can eat for your microbiome to boost the "good" bacteria and not feed the "bad" bacteria. They are as follows.

Eat a High-Fiber Diet

A high-fiber diet can help decrease the inflammation associated with leaky gut syndrome. Here's how Marcelo Campos, MD, a primary care doctor at Harvard Vanguard, explained leaky gut: "Inside our bellies, we have an extensive intestinal lining covering more than 4,000 square feet of surface area. When working properly, it forms a tight barrier that controls what gets absorbed into the bloodstream. An unhealthy gut lining may have large cracks or holes, allowing partially digested food, toxins, and bugs to penetrate the tissues beneath it. This may trigger inflammation and changes in the gut flora (normal bacteria) that could lead to problems within the digestive tract and beyond." If you have gastrointestinal distress, ulcers, gas or bloating, diarrhea, gastroesophageal reflux disease (GERD), heartburn, or indigestion, it could be related to leaky gut, and consuming more fiber can help.

A high-fiber diet also seems to help the body process estrogen. "When a high-fiber diet is consumed, the estrobolome increases the metabolism of estrogen and thus its elimination from the body," the Kaiser Permanente researchers wrote. "Because nearly 70 percent of breast cancers are estrogen fueled, a high-fiber diet contributes to estrogen elimination, robbing breast cancer cells of a major fuel source. The 'commonsense' recommendation to increase dietary fiber in the setting of breast cancer decreases inflammation. The increased consumption of fiber and polyphenols"—powerful antioxidants—"readily available from a whole-food, plant-based diet, contributes to an overall increase in breast cancer survival."

There are two types of fiber: soluble, found in wheat bran, beans, whole grains, and seeds, which pulls in water, slows digestion, and lowers cholesterol levels; and insoluble, found in fruits and vegetables, as well as whole grains and wheat bran, which helps speed up digestion and move stool. Fiber also helps feed the good bacteria in your system—so-called prebiotics. Getting a mix of fiber from lots of sources ensures that you maximize your nutritional load. Some of my favorites are barley; buckwheat noodles; cruciferous vegetables such as Brussels sprouts, broccoli, and watercress; yuca; Chinese cabbage; daikon; lentils; avocados; nuts and seeds such as sunflower, pistachios, and walnuts; figs; berries; apples; quinoa; and popcorn. Aim to get at least 25 grams of fiber a day. For reference, a baked potato with skin has 4 grams of fiber, a cup of whole wheat spaghetti has 6 grams of fiber, and 1 ounce of chia seeds has 10 grams of fiber.

Focus on Fermented Foods

These foods contain probiotics, which are "good" bacteria. They include kimchi, miso, sauerkraut, kefir, tempeh, and kombucha.

CHAPTER 10

Body Movement
for Menopause

What's your favorite way to move your body? Do you like to run or jog? Is Zumba or dance class your thing? Are you a yoga and Pilates kind of person? Are you on the tennis court five days a week? Whatever your answer to that question is, *I love it!* If you're not doing something that brings you happiness, you won't do it consistently.

In other parts of the book, I talked about the value of cardio, yoga, and exercising in nature. But I can't talk about body movement for menopause without touching on weight training. Doing movements that pound on the body—think jogging, skipping rope, playing pickleball or basketball—as well as lifting weights creates microtears in the bones, which then grow back stronger. It's the same way that muscles get stronger.

There's another advantage to weight training that to me is just as important. It makes you feel like a total badass. I spoke with Dianna Scotece, CSCS, a New York–based strength coach who specializes in training women over fifty, as well as utilizing lifting as a way to cope with trauma. Scotece competed in Olympic weight lifting for more than ten years, and when other women saw her training in the gym, they asked if she could train them, too. "Something started happening with women doing shoulder presses, kettlebell swings, back squats, bench presses, deadlifts—these women who had raised kids, put themselves through school, were close to retiring. They felt newly empowered by lifting. They experienced a difference in their body confidence, in their gym confidence," she told me.

I asked Scotece what makes weight training so powerful for people who have never done it before. Her response really hit me: you end up learning that a part of you exists that you're discovering for the first time. "It's like finding out you had a whole extra bedroom in your apartment," she said. "Many people get told they don't belong here. In the gym. In other places they want to be. They were told they shouldn't even *be* who they wanted to be. This is an opportunity to go somewhere you were told you don't belong. Imagine that time you were not allowed to go somewhere. Now imagine walking through that door."

That's why Scotece works with Sanctuary for Families, an organization in New York that provides service and advocacy for women, transgender, and nonbinary survivors of domestic violence, sex trafficking, and related forms of gender violence as well as their families. There's emerging research into using strength training as a tool of recovery from domestic violence, and Scotece teaches survivor leaders how to teach weight lifting so they can share it with others. She told me about a survivor client who broke down and cried because the lifting had dredged up their past in a painful way. "Until then, they didn't know they could rely on their body," Scotece said. "How fucked up is that? Someone had denied them access to their body." Fittingly, Scotece is founding her own nonprofit, Muscle Inspires New Empowerment (MINE).

If you're starting your lifting journey during the menopausal transition, that's wonderful! A great way to find consistency and peace is to get real with what you want out of it. Do you want to find a community? Are you looking for self-sufficiency? (When you buy a thirty-pound bag of dog food and decline the offer from the seventeen-year-old to carry it out to your car for you, throw it over your shoulder, and carry it yourself, that's what you call a power move.) Do you want to explore your body more deeply, especially in this time of so much change? Do you want to feel what it's like to stand in front of a heavy and daunting barbell, pick it up, and put it back down with pride? "One other draw is for people who've gone through shit. People who have learned the value of life," Scotece told me. "People who have been through it but retained the innocence of curiosity, entering the gym with a sense of wonder." And who hasn't been through some shit in their life? Beloved family members die. Families fall apart. Friends get sick. Jobs are lost. I don't need to list all the ways in which bad things can and do happen. There are a lot of ways we can cope with bad things. Finding peace in the gym is one of the healthier options.

My goal for everyone is that they move their body every day, ideally for at least thirty minutes. You're not going to be hulking out every day! I can't make a recommendation that is one size fits all, but what I can say is that your week should be a mix of activities that build muscle and bone (weight lifting, doing bodyweight exercises, doing pounding movements such as jumping rope), get your heart rate up (short and brisk jogging, shadow boxing, doing a fast swim, rowing, dancing), work on your endurance (taking a long walk, doing a long slow swim, shooting hoops, doing upper body resistance band work), and help with active recovery (doing yoga or tai chi). Find the mix that's right for you! Remember our mantra: consistency and peace. It might take some time, even six months or a year, to find the right mix for you. Here's how I think about it: Exercise should empty your cup because you're working hard, but it should fill your cup up again with what it gives back to you and how it makes you feel. As you progress, the amount you have to give as well as the amount you get back will increase. That's how capacity, strength, and power build over time.

The research is pretty irrefutable that some sort of resistance work is really important for the menopausal transition and beyond, both physically and psychologically. For the uninitiated, weight training does require some know-how, so it's important to find someone who can guide you and watch your form. You can find that through:

- A personal trainer who specializes in working with people in their forties plus, particularly people who are going through the menopausal transition (the personal training director at your gym can help identify the right person for you)
- An online personal trainer, which tends to be more affordable than an in-person trainer and who can respond to your body's needs, including adaptive weight training for people who have different abilities, before or after a treatment or surgery such as mastectomy or hysterectomy, or helping heal an injury
- Group fitness classes at the YMCA, JCC, or local rec center
- Specialty lifting gyms that have programming especially for those in their forties
- An online community for lifting and exercising that works for you, such as The Queer Gym (https://www.thequeergym.com/)

Regardless of your age, you have to enter this process in communication with your body. Working out is uncomfortable, but there's a difference between discomfort and pain. Some days your body will be raring to go, and other days you just won't have enough juice. If you're chronically tired and sleeping doesn't restore your pep, my next question would be whether you're eating enough. Many of us equate working out with losing weight or changing the aesthetics of our appearance. That's often related to the body dysmorphia many of us have related to eating. *We should not apologize or try to atone for our bodies. We should not apologize or atone for the natural changes our bodies go through.* Remember what Robyn Goldberg said: that our body's metabolism slows for a reason. It enables extra fat to accumulate, and that fat stores estrogen that helps save our bones and keeps all of the systems that get a kick out of hormones running better. As a doctor, am I still worried about some of the diseases that medicine traditionally associates with carrying more weight? Yes. But the solution *isn't* to measure your weight changes. As discussed in part II, we need to look at the other, more accurate, metrics: blood sugar and A1C levels; blood pressure, resting heart rate, and heart rate variability; inflammation markers; circulating cholesterol levels. Those numbers, plus learning from you about how you're feeling, will tell me way more than a scale ever will.

You Don't Have to Get Weighed at the Doctor's

In case no one has ever told you, having your weight checked at the doctor's office isn't required. Unless you've experienced a huge weight swing (which might indicate an underlying disease), there's not much to be learned from your weight. Of course, there are times when a doctor needs your accurate weight; for instance, an anesthesiologist needs it if you're going in for surgery, and some treatments are mass specific.

Here are the benefits of not being weighed. One, your doctor doesn't make a snap judgment about you. It is well documented that physicians see the weight of a patient and attribute whatever ailments they have to their size. I couldn't find hard data on this, but there are likely tens of thousands or more women whose cancers or other diseases have been missed or diagnosed late because their physician said their symptoms were because they were fat and if they weren't fat, they wouldn't be sick. The thought makes me shudder. The other benefit of declining being weighed is that it makes the patient feel better. Some people have such a visceral negative reaction to being weighed and having their weight made public that they don't go to the doctor. Or they say that it's the most stressful part of a doctor's appointment. If that's the case, *just say no!* Politely decline. Say, "I'd prefer not to get weighed." Or ask the physician assistant or nurse practitioner why they need your weight. If they truly need it and it's not just a box in an intake form they're filling in, you can do a "blind weighing": stand facing away from the scale, and ask the person weighing you not to say the number aloud.

Until we decouple what we weigh from our feelings of self-worth, the scale will always have too much power over us. Using the scale on only a few occasions is a good stopgap measure.

The other reason you might be overly fatigued, particularly when you've just started on your fitness journey, is that you haven't given your body enough time to rest. Athletes and weekend warriors alike have to get into tune with their body so they know when to give it a break and how. Gregory Alan Reid, a longtime trainer and pro body-builder in Los Angeles, says that downtime is essential for the body to repair itself. "Without proper downtime, counting rest and sleep, the body is not going to grow right," he told me. He also talked about this in terms of vibration: sometimes you're vibrating at a high fre-quency and need to bring it down. Try using a foam roller or physio balls to slowly stretch out your muscles. That kind of stretching is great for your tendons, joints, and muscles, bringing circulation "to all the nooks and crannies of the body," he told me.

Most people think about stretching before and after they work out, but try to add a stretching routine before bed, as well. Think about it this way: the entire day of running around, sitting at your desk, cooking, running errands, having a walk and talk with a friend is like working out! You want to make all your muscles and joints supple and relaxed so you can get a body-stress-free sleep. Spend ten or fifteen minutes foam rolling your glutes, shoulder blades, hip flexors, and anywhere else that has tightness. Use a golf ball to stretch out the bottoms of your feet. Use a percussive massage device, such as a Theragun, to thump the big muscles. Try it for about two weeks, and see if you sleep better.

CHAPTER 11

Consider Botanical
Supplements

By the time you're this far into *Menopause Bootcamp*, you'll have understood that my approach to this time of life is *whatever works best for you*. For a lot of my patients, that *might* include taking supplements. I say "might" because, like everything else, it's highly personal. Here's the thing: I have no accurate way of predicting which of the panoply of supplements will be effective for your system. Going the supplement route will inevitably involve trying something for three to six months and, if it's not giving you the desired result, moving onto something else. That may sound like a bummer. After all, we're used to taking a drug and having it work more or less immediately, as well as having strict guidelines and FDA approvals that pair drugs with the conditions they treat. To embark on botanical supplements, it's helpful to approach the process with curiosity and flexibility.

The list below is meant to be user friendly, organized by the experience you'd like to ameliorate or enhance. *Use only one supplement per symptom at any one time*—meaning that if you want to address hot flashes, for example, take only one supplement for hot flashes. Please be careful about the brands that you buy. I have listed my preferred purveyors of each supplement. I've carefully chosen them because the origin of their products is safe, the contents on the label accurately reflect what's in the bottle, and, in the case of Kindra and Enzymedica, I know the company leadership and trust their processes.

If you have a preexisting medical condition, please consult your physician before taking any of these. Of course, if you take a supplement and you start to feel unwell, discontinue taking it immediately. If you feel quite ill or as though you're having an allergic reaction, call your physician or, in an emergency, dial 911. I have never, ever had that experience in my practice with any of the supplements listed below. But you can never be too careful!

Mountain Rose Herbs is a wonderful source of herbs, botanicals, recipes, and resources. One other herbal supplement I would like to share with you is a special tea blend created by Mary Thompson, one of my Ayurvedic mentors. "The Rasa tea is a nourishing tea that helps build all the vital fluids of the body. This will help with hydration as well as circulation of the blood and support proper functioning of all body organs and systems. Your skin will be moister and your whole body cooler when you incorporate this tea on a regular basis," Thompson says.

How to Make Mary's Rasa Tea

Into a large pot, place ¼ cup each fennel seeds, fenugreek seeds, licorice bark, and cinnamon bark. Add 4 cups of water. Bring to a boil over medium heat, then remove, cover, and let steep for at least 30 minutes. Strain out the herbs, refrigerate when the tea is at room temperature, and drink a small cup daily.

Substitutions and modifications:

In place of/in addition to fennel: anise, grated fresh ginger

In place of/in addition to fenugreek: burdock root, Indian sarsa-parilla

In place of/in addition to licorice bark: shatavari, marshmallow root

In place of/in addition to cinnamon bark: cardamom seeds, ginger

Herb/ Supplement	What It Is For	Dosage	What You Should Know	Brand Name/ Manufacturer
Berberine	Improvement of insulin level, glucose level, metabolism; weight loss	Follow dosage directions on packaging	Do not take if you have kidney disease	Enzymedica
Cinnamon	Improvement of insulin level, glucose level, metabolism; weight loss	420 mg per day	Must use the supplement, not the kitchen spice. And do not exceed this dosage.	Mountain Rose Herbs
Maitake mushroom extract	Improvement of metabolism	50 mg per day		Mountain Rose Herbs
Inositol	Improvement of metabolism	400 mg three times a day, not to exceed four months' duration	Do not take if you have kidney or liver disease	Metagenic
Ashwagandha	Improvement of mood; alleviation of stress	500 mg three times a day, not to exceed 6 g per day	Do not take if you have thyroid disease	Banyan Botanicals
Shatavari	Improvement of mood; alleviation of stress	Follow dosage directions on packaging	Do not take if you have estrogen-dependent cancers	Banyan Botanicals
5HTP	Improvement of mood; alleviation of stress	100–300 mg three times a day	Do not take if you are on an SSRI or tramadol	Metagenics
Holy basil (tulsi) tincture	Alleviation of stress; improvement of energy; lessening of fatigue	2–3 mL per day		Banyan Botanicals
Rhodiola	Improvement of mood; alleviation of stress	200-400 mg per day		Mountain Rose Herbs
Passionflower	Improvement of mood, sleep; alleviation of stress	320 mg at bedtime or three times a day		Mountain Rose Herbs
Lion's mane mushrooms	Improvement of mood, cognition; alleviation of anxiety	Follow dosage directions on packaging	Do not take if you have asthma or allergies	Mountain Rose Herbs

Herb/ Supplement	What It Is For	Dosage	What You Should Know	Brand Name/ Manufacturer
Maca root powder	Alleviation of stress; improvement of mood, energy, libido	75–100 mg per day or 3 g per day in a smoothie		Mountain Rose Herbs
D-mannose	Prevention of urinary tract symptoms	500 mg two times a day		Ellura (its formula also contains cranberry)
Cranberry extract	Prevention of urinary tract symptoms	Follow dosage directions on packaging		Mountain Rose Herbs
Diindolylmethane (DIM)	Overall estrogen dominance; well-being	100–200 mg per day	Do not take if you have liver or kidney disease	Metagenics
Indole-3-carbinol (alternative for DIM)	Overall estrogen dominance; well-being	250–600 mg per day	Do not take if you have liver or kidney disease	Metagenics
Vitex/chaste tree berry	Overall estrogen dominance; improvement of PMS; possibly alleviation of hot flashes	Use as directed; depends on brand		Vital Nutrients, Vitex 750
Russian raspberry	Alleviation of hot flashes	Follow dosage directions on packaging	Do not take if you have estrogen-dependent cancers	Metagenics, Estrovera
Black cohosh	Alleviation of hot flashes	20 mg two times per day		Remifemin
Pycnogenol/ French marine pine bark extract	Alleviation of hot flashes	Follow dosage directions on packaging		Kindra Core Support
Nettle infuswion/tea	Hair loss			Mountain Rose Herbs
CBD/CBN	Alleviation of anxiety; improvement of mood, sleep, sexual health	Follow dosage directions on packaging		Cannapy Health
Hair wellness blend	Hair loss	Follow dosage directions on packaging	Do not take if you have estrogen-dependent cancers	Nutrafol

CHAPTER 12

Build Your Team, Be a Good Teammate

In the tennis legend Andre Agassi's memoir *Open*, he wrote extensively about his team. It comprises his longtime trainer and father figure, Gil Reyes; his caring brother, Phillip; Brad Gilbert, the coach who first believed in him; and his compassionate wife, Stefanie Graf, a world-class tennis player herself. That team was steadfast. They celebrated his glorious wins, and they scraped him off the floor after his heart-wrenching losses—and worse. Don't we all deserve a team like that? An all-star team is one that gives us the ability to try to achieve big things and take risks. They will celebrate our glorious wins and help us through our heart-wrenching losses. They will love us for our flaws, not in spite of them.

A good teammate for you might be a therapist or other mental health professional. The stigma of poor mental health seems to be eroding, but it's still out there. If you think you might want to establish a relationship with a mental health professional, do it. Here's how I think about it: People inevitably go through tough times in their lives. And it's easier to have an established relationship with someone so they're not meeting you for the first time when you're in crisis. Telemedicine has become widely available for mental health care, so it's easier than ever to find someone who aligns with your needs, especially if you're a member of a marginalized community.

Getting your head straight is important. But a therapist sees you only so often. Whom do you interact with in your day-to-day life? A partner, family members, friends, work colleagues, fitness professionals, and members of a faith community, club, or volunteer organization—they can all be on your team. One thing I've found is that people who traverse the menopausal transition with the most psychic ease do so because of having the support of at least a few close people. The same goes for a major medical event. Find the people who are constants, who bring you peace.

And be a good teammate. I swear, if there is one thing that seems to be a cure-all when you're feeling bad, it's being of service to others. When you look for ways to do good, you break down your ego in a Freudian sense. You counteract the worldview that puts you at the center. Seeing the needs of others and responding to them gives you a sense of wholeness that you may not be able to achieve if you act only in service to yourself. It's as I said at the beginning of the section: almost all healthy relationships require both input and output. You are beaming your energy to another person; they are beaming their energy to you.

At this point I have a favor to ask. The book you have in your hands is just that—a collection of pages, information, mantras, reframing, and the like. Some of it has spoken to you, I hope; some of it hasn't. The reason it is so broad is that the goal is erecting a big tent, a Kevlar-strong, multicolored, climate-controlled tent that *everyone* will view as a safe space. We cannot be of service to others unless we are curious and compassionate about the people who are not like us. We cannot live a full life unless we are of service to others.

Here goes my big ask: Will you be the founder of your own Menopause Bootcamp? It's a little daunting, I know, but the rewards can be life changing. Getting started is as easy as contacting a few close pals and having each one contact one more person, each of whom is somewhere along the menopause journey. Get together for an hour, socially distanced and outdoors if need be—and snacks are always helpful. Don't forget to hydrate! Share a few of the things that you've learned. Reflect on what you've read and how it connects to you. Invite others to open up, too.

I don't want to ruin the surprise, but I want to entice you into doing this by telling you about the beautiful things that will happen. People are squeamish in the beginning. Seldom are we invited to talk about this life event; when we do, we are so often made to feel bad. Watching a group of people go from anxiety to relief and being the agent of that metamorphosis is the most incredible thing. You see their postures change. They go from being scrunched up to sitting tall, shoulders back. They exude openness. You see them go from breathing shallowly and holding in their bellies—signs of stress and a desire to conform—to breathing big, laughing loudly, and releasing their bodies to own their space. What happens next is incredible: they take all that beautiful energy and reinvigorated spirit and *share it with others*. They replace judgment with curiosity, ego with service, shame with pride. All of that makes us powerful. This is why the patriarchy wants to keep us uncomfortable and defensive. When we're together, fully living in our bodies, that is when we get shit done.

CHAPTER 13

Start a Menopause Bootcamp

Here's the beauty of the book you're reading. Most all of the insights I have as a physician and Ayurvedic practitioner are contained in these pages. Of course, there's a different dynamic in person; it's technicolor rather than black and white. But my presence isn't the thing that makes Menopause Bootcamp sessions come to life—it's the collective. My recommendation would be to invite a group to meet once a month for four months. All of the participants could get a copy of this book or designate one to be the go-to person for the info. Each meeting can focus on one part. Here are some ideas.

- Start with a short guided meditation or guided breathwork (you can use an app). This quiet moment of reflection designates a distinct starting point for the bootcamp, helping to separate it from whatever's going on in the other parts of your life. Use this time to set ground rules: what is said here stays here, boundaries are respected, and creating a safe space is tantamount.

◆ During the first session, even if people already know one another, go around and introduce yourselves, say why you decided to join, and offer one fact about yourself. Sharing is *not* compulsory. Some people need to warm up to the process.

◆ After that, and in subsequent sessions, use one of the conversation starters below to instigate sharing and create the safe environment that's a hallmark of the Menopause Bootcamp.

◆ Go over the part of the book designated for that month. Talk about some of the overall learnings from that section, along with actionable suggestions. Invite conversations about people's experiences, what has worked for them and what hasn't, and workshop ideas to help those gathered integrate some of the suggestions from this book into their own lives.

◆ Spend ten to fifteen minutes talking about self-acceptance and creating trust. These conversations can imprint themselves on people's hearts.

◆ If it's within your capabilities, invite a bodywork specialist, such as a yoga instructor or personal trainer, to lead the group through moves that work the core, focusing on form, function, and everyday movements. An online leader works great for this, either something that's prerecorded or done live for your group.

◆ In closing, go around the group and invite the participants to say one bit of information they learned, an action item they want to try, and one thing they're grateful for. Thank everyone for their generosity of spirit. A post–Menopause Bootcamp lunch is always fun, too.

After the four initial sessions, feel free to meet as often as feels good. Use the conversation starters to go into deeper discussions. Brainstorm ways in which you can help others going through the menopausal transition, including volunteering your time or educating yourself about the experiences of others in different countries or communities. If your participation in the bootcamp was powerful, consider forming a new group to share information from the book and learnings from your friends.

Twelve Conversation Starters

1. Are there people in your life you want to share your experience with but don't feel you can? What is stopping you? How can you overcome the barrier?

2. What are you most looking forward to in menopause?

3. Does menopause impact you at work? What could your workplace do to make things better for you?

4. For many, menopause is a time of liberation. What are you feeling liberated from?

5. Who is your postmenopause icon? Whose power do you emulate?

6. Would you like to talk about your sex life or self-pleasure? What's working for you these days?

7. When you're feeling really good, how do you channel your good vibes? What about when you're feeling down? How do you lift yourself out of that place?

8. How has covid-19 made you change the way you see yourself in the world?

9. Is there something that's stopping you from living the kind of life you want to? Are there things your family and friends can do to take down those barriers?

10. When something goes awry in your life—menopause related or not—do you have ways to ask for help?

11. How do you see yourself one, five, and ten years from now? What priorities does your future vision embody? Freedom? Adventure? Serenity? Love? Health?

12. How can you reach out to others not in your immediate circle or community to support them through their menopause journey?

You are now officially a graduate of the Menopause Bootcamp! I challenge you to say the word *menopause* out loud often—often enough that you don't even notice the taboo you are slowly chipping away at. Know that you are part of a tribe that is as ancient, mysteriously enchanting, and powerful as the hills. The power derives from the confidence of your experiences and the willingness to share who you really are with yourself and a world that desperately needs loving wisdom. I hope you take great care in getting to know this part of yourself, as much as you would a new friend, lover, or member of your inner circle. I hope you realize how honored I am to serve her and watch her evolve. I hope you understand that I learn from her just as much as I have shared.

ACKNOWLEDGMENTS

My childhood dream was to be an author and it goes without saying that I absolutely would not be here offering you all this book without an enormous, active, creative, talented, and generous village to support and guide me through this process. But I'll go ahead and say it anyway, because apparently that is what authors do, and now I am an author.

Thank you to every patient, student, and TV producer who asked, "Where is your book?" and inspired me to just do it already.

Thank you to my team at UTA who believed in me and in this project for longer than I did: Brandi Bowles, Ennis Kamcile, and Ryan Hayden. Thank you to Yasmeen Al-shawwa for keeping me on task and sharing my vision. Thank you to Karen Rinaldi and Rachel Kambury and everyone at Harper Wave for getting this project and getting me.

Thank you to my mentors and colleagues Dr. Mark Tager, Dr. Micheal Krychman, Dr. Jane Van Dis, all the incredible women physicians in the OMG group, and to my partners, staff, and coworkers at Women's Care of Beverly Hills, but especially to Cathy Moraga and

Jackey Morando for putting up with me day in and day out—and to Judy Ervin and Sherrie Barnes for being sounding boards. Thank you to Dr. Marc Halpern, Arun Deva, Mary Thompson, and generations of Ayurvedic teachers and practitioners before them, and thank you to Dorit Dyke who brought this lineage to me.

There would not be a book were it not for Marjorie Korn's capacity to see the forest for the trees and then take the pruning shears to those trees in order to forge an actual walkable path. Thank you for co-piloting this project.

Thank you to the numerous experts who agreed to discuss this evolving topic and share their experience, research, and insights: Mary Thompson; Robyn Goldberg, RDN; CERD-S; Dr. Suzanne Steinbaum; Maurice Garcia, MD; Emeran Mayer, MD; Mona Eltahawy; Meg Bradbury; Denise Pines; Jolinda Johnson; Sarah Hill, PhD; Dianna Scotece, CSCS.

Thank you to my kids, Jaron and Georgia Lenz, for the opportunity to be and grow into the mom I am, for keeping it real even when I don't enjoy it, for tolerating my endless curiosity, submitting themselves as experimental subjects for all my remedy preparations. Thank you to my dad, Dr. Arny Gilberg, the OG outside-the-box thinker who raised me to do the right thing even when others didn't understand what I was doing, and whose endless kvelling about his daughter, the doctor, means so much. A bittersweet thanks to my mom, Lynne, who was always my biggest cheerleader. She passed away just after this book was accepted for publication but didn't live to read how much her insistence on my being independent resulted in this work. She would have been so proud.

Thank you to Jay Gilberg, whose integrity and unconditional support has sustained me since we met when I was eighteen months old. I'm sorry I tried to suffocate you as an infant; you turned out to be an outstanding man and brother.

Thank you to all of my patients and the participants in Menopause

Bootcamp for inspiring me to create this opportunity for all of us to live here and now and grow every day. Thank you for trusting me, sharing with me, and supporting me.

Thank you to my dear friends Rebecca Benenati for seeing the value in hosting and promoting MBC, and Erica Chidi for asking the right questions at the exact right times. And to my "sisters," Tracey Pepper, Deanna Noe, Sophia Grant, Rona Heifetz, Cynthia Willard, and Jennifer Trilling, I am forever in gratitude.

Last, to my life partner and love, Greg Reid. You are my redwood tree, truly sheltering me through every storm and being the light that illuminates my journey. You have continued to push me ever deeper into understanding and loving the me that I share with all of you while simultaneously standing right next to me in solidarity.

NOTES

Introduction

xvi A 2013 survey: Christianson, M. S., Ducie, J. A., Altman, K., Khafagy, A. M., & Shen, W. (2013). Menopause education. *Menopause, 20*(11), 1120–1125. https://doi.org/10.1097/gme.0b013e31828ced7f

Chapter 1: The Basics

7 as the number of women: Bui, Q., & Miller, C. C. (2018, August 4). The age that women have babies: How a gap divides America. *The New York Times.* https://www.nytimes.com/interactive/2018/08/04/upshot/up-birth-age-gap.html

8 Psoriasis is a skin condition: Ceovic, R., Mance, M., Bukvic Mokos, Z., Svetec, M., Kostovic, K., & Stulhofer Buzina, D. (2013). Psoriasis: Female skin changes in various hormonal stages throughout life—puberty, pregnancy, and menopause. *BioMed Research International, 2013*, Article 571912. https://doi.org/10.1155/2013/571912

13 and therefore hadn't breastfed: National Cancer Institute. (n.d.). *Reproductive history and cancer risk.* https://www.cancer.gov/about-cancer/causes-prevention/risk/hormones/reproductive-history-fact-sheet

13 For context, a survey: Mirza, S. A., & Rooney, C. (2019, July 19). *Discrimination prevents LGBTQ people from accessing health care.* Center for American Progress. https://americanprogress.org/article/discrimination-prevents-lgbtq-people-accessing-health-care/

14 some studies suggest: Cleveland Clinic. (n.d.). *Spontaneous coronary artery dissection (SCAD).* https://my.clevelandclinic.org/health/diseases/17503-spontaneous-coronary-artery-dissection-scad

Chapter 2: Hormones and "The Big Four"

19 micronized progesterone: Asi, N., Mohammed, K., Haydour, Q., Gionfriddo, M. R., Vargas, O. L., Prokop, L. J., Faubion, S. S., & Murad, M. H. (2016). Progesterone vs. synthetic progestins and the risk of breast

cancer: A systematic review and meta-analysis. *Systematic Reviews, 5*(1). https://doi.org/10.1186/s13643-016-0294-5

22   *subclinical hypothyroidism*: Kim, Y. A., & Park, Y. J. (2014). Prevalence and risk factors of subclinical thyroid disease. *Endocrinology and Metabolism, 29*(1), 20. https://doi.org/10.3803/enm.2014.29.1.20

27   If she has a unilateral oophorectomy: Rosendahl, M., Simonsen, M. K., & Kjer, J. J. (2017). The influence of unilateral oophorectomy on the age of menopause. *Climacteric, 20*(6), 540–544. https://doi.org/10.1080/136 97137.2017.1369512

Chapter 3: The Symptoms of Menopause

43   For most people: Freedman, R. R. (2014). Menopausal hot flashes: Mechanisms, endocrinology, treatment. *The Journal of Steroid Biochemistry and Molecular Biology, 142*, 115–120. https://doi.org/10.1016/j.jsbmb.2013 .08.010

44   Researchers from Liverpool John Moores University: Freedman, R. R. (2014). Menopausal hot flashes: Mechanisms, endocrinology, treatment. *The Journal of Steroid Biochemistry and Molecular Biology, 142*, 115–120. https://doi.org/10.1016/j.jsbmb.2013.08.010

45   A 2021 paper: Thurston, R. C., Aslanidou Vlachos, H. E., Derby, C. A., Jackson, E. A., Brooks, M. M., Matthews, K. A., Harlow, S., Joffe, H., & El Khoudary, S. R. (2021). Menopausal vasomotor symptoms and risk of incident cardiovascular disease events in Swan. *Journal of the American Heart Association, 10*(3), Article e017416. https://doi.org/10.1161/jaha .120.017416

48   The evidence on bias: Wright, K. (2021, July 21). *Opinion: Gender bias in the OR is a hazard to patient safety*. MedPage Today. https://www.medpage today.com/opinion/second-opinions/93685

49   In the absence of research: Thurston, R. C., Aslanidou Vlachos, H. E., Derby, C. A., Jackson, E. A., Brooks, M. M., Matthews, K. A., Harlow, S., Joffe, H., & El Khoudary, S. R. (2021). Menopausal vasomotor symptoms and risk of incident cardiovascular disease events in Swan. *Journal of the American Heart Association, 10*(3). https://doi.org/10.1161/jaha .120.017416

50   "The under-representation of women": Brazil, R. (2020, May 28). Why we need to talk about sex and clinical trials. *The Pharmaceutical Journal.* https://pharmaceutical-journal.com/article/feature/why-we-need-to-talk -about-sex-and-clinical-trials

50   2020 review: Brazil, R. (2020, May 28). Why we need to talk about sex and clinical trials. *The Pharmaceutical Journal.* https://pharmaceutical -journal.com/article/feature/why-we-need-to-talk-about-sex-and-clinical -trials

52 Women's Health Initiative: Writing Group for the Women's Health Initiative Investigators. (2002). Risks and benefits of estrogen plus progestin in healthy postmenopausal women: Principal results from the Women's Health Initiative Randomized Controlled Trial. *JAMA: The Journal of the American Medical Association, 288*(3), 321–333. https://doi.org/10.1001/jama.288.3.321

55 "The term *bioidentical hormone*": Files, J. A., Ko, M. G., & Pruthi, S. (2011). Bioidentical hormone therapy. *Mayo Clinic Proceedings, 86*(7), 673–680. https://doi.org/10.4065/mcp.2010.0714

55 American College of Obstetricians and Gynecologists: American College of Obstetricians and Gynecologists. (n.d.). *Compounded bioidentical menopausal hormone therapy.* https://www.acog.org/clinical/clinical -guidance/committee-opinion/articles/2012/08/compounded-bioidentical -menopausal-hormone-therapy

55 Endocrine Society: Santoro, N., Braunstein, G. D., Butts, C. L., Martin, K. A., McDermott, M., & Pinkerton, J. A. V. (2016). Compounded bioidentical hormones in endocrinology practice: An endocrine society scientific statement. *The Journal of Clinical Endocrinology & Metabolism, 101*(4), 1318–1343. https://doi.org/10.1210/jc.2016-1271

57 a 2017 study: Thompson, J. J., Ritenbaugh, C., & Nichter, M. (2017). Why women choose compounded bioidentical hormone therapy: Lessons from a qualitative study of menopausal decision-making. *BMC Women's Health, 17*(1). https://doi.org/10.1186/s12905-017-0449-0

58 the first FDA-approved estrogen product: American College of Obstetricians and Gynecologists. (n.d.). *Compounded bioidentical menopausal hormone therapy.* https://www.acog.org/clinical/clinical-guidance /committee-opinion/articles/2012/08/compounded-bioidentical -menopausal-hormone-therapy

61 A review of research: Shams, T., Firwana, B., Habib, F., Alshahrani, A., AlNouh, B., Murad, M. H., & Ferwana, M. (2013). SSRIs for hot flashes: A systematic review and meta-analysis of randomized trials. *Journal of General Internal Medicine, 29*(1), 204–213. https://doi.org/10.1007/s11606-013-2535-9

61 They may not be good: Stubbs, C., Mattingly, L., Crawford, S. A., Wickersham, E. A., Brockhaus, J. L., & McCarthy, L. H. (2017, May). Do SSRIs and SNRIs reduce the frequency and/or severity of hot flashes in menopausal women. *The Journal of the Oklahoma State Medical Association.* https://www.ncbi.nlm.nih.gov/pmc/articles/PMC5482277/

63 it may change the efficacy: Asher, G. N., Corbett, A. H., & Hawke, R. L. (2017, July 15). Common herbal dietary supplement-drug interactions. *American Family Physician.* https://www.aafp.org/afp/2017/0715/p101 .html

63 Red clover's effectiveness: Ghazanfarpour, M., Sadeghi, R., Roudsari,

R. L., Khorsand, I., Khadivzadeh, T., & Muoio, B. (2015). Red clover for treatment of hot flashes and menopausal symptoms: A systematic review and meta-analysis. *Journal of Obstetrics and Gynaecology*, *36*(3), 301–311. https://doi.org/10.3109/01443615.2015.1049249

63 It's available in: Icahn School of Medicine at Mount Sinai. (n.d.). *Red clover*. https://www.mountsinai.org/health-library/herb/red-clover

63 A 2019 paper: Pabich, M., & Materska, M. (2019). Biological effect of soy isoflavones in the prevention of civilization diseases. *Nutrients*, *11*(7), 1660. https://doi.org/10.3390/nu11071660

63 The data are mostly inconclusive: Lethaby, A., Marjoribanks, J., Kronenberg, F., Roberts, H., Eden, J., & Brown, J. (2013). *Phytoestrogens for menopausal vasomotor symptoms*. Cochrane Database of Systematic Reviews. https://doi.org/10.1002/14651858.cd001395.pub4

64 potent anticancer benefits: Basu, P., & Maier, C. (2018). Phytoestrogens and breast cancer: In vitro anticancer activities of isoflavones, lignans, coumestans, stilbenes and their analogs and derivatives. *Biomedicine & Pharmacotherapy*, *107*, 1648–1666. https://doi.org/10.1016/j.biopha.2018.08.100

64 "While there is no clear evidence": Fritz, H., Seely, D., Flower, G., Skidmore, B., Fernandes, R., Vadeboncoeur, S., Kennedy, D., Cooley, K., Wong, R., Sagar, S., Sabri, E., & Fergusson, D. (2013). Soy, red clover, and isoflavones and breast cancer: A systematic review. *PLoS ONE*, *8*(11). https://doi.org/10.1371/journal.pone.0081968

64 In some small randomized trials: Kazemi, F., Masoumi, S. Z., Shayan, A., & Oshvandi, K. (2021). The effect of evening primrose oil capsule on hot flashes and night sweats in postmenopausal women: A single-blind randomized controlled trial. *Journal of Menopausal Medicine*, *27*(1), 8. https://doi.org/10.6118/jmm.20033

64 according to a paper: Vollmer, G., Papke, A., & Zierau, O. (2010). Treatment of menopausal symptoms by an extract from the roots of rhapontic rhubarb: The role of estrogen receptors. *Chinese Medicine*, *5*(1), 7. https://doi.org/10.1186/1749-8546-5-7

65 cardiometabolic: Malekahmadi, M., Moradi Moghaddam, O., Firouzi, S., Daryabeygi-Khotbehsara, R., Shariful Islam, S. M., Norouzy, A., & Soltani, S. (2019). Effects of pycnogenol on cardiometabolic health: A systematic review and meta-analysis of randomized controlled trials. *Pharmacological Research*, *150*, Article 104472. https://doi.org/10.1016/j.phrs.2019.104472

65 brain health: Malekahmadi, M., Moradi Moghaddam, O., Firouzi, S., Daryabeygi-Khotbehsara, R., Shariful Islam, S. M., Norouzy, A., & Soltani, S. (2019). Effects of pycnogenol on cardiometabolic health: A systematic review and meta-analysis of randomized controlled trials. *Phar-*

macological Research, 150, Article 104472. https://doi.org/10.1016
/j.phrs.2019.104472

65 in addition to hot flashes: Yang, H.-M., Liao, M.-F., Zhu, S.-Y., Liao,
M.-N., & Rohdewald, P. (2007). A randomised, double-blind, placebo-
controlled trial on the effect of Pycnogenol® on the climacteric syndrome
in peri-menopausal women. *Acta Obstetricia et Gynecologica Scandinavica,*
86(8), 978–985. https://doi.org/10.1080/00016340701446108

65 treatment of osteoporosis: Kim, J.-L., Kim, Y.-H., Kang, M.-K., Gong,
J.-H., Han, S.-J., & Kang, Y.-H. (2013). Antiosteoclastic activity of milk
thistle extract after ovariectomy to suppress estrogen deficiency-induced
osteoporosis. *BioMed Research International, 2013,* Article 919374.
https://doi.org/10.1155/2013/919374

65 reduction of hot flashes: Saberi, Z., Gorji, N., Memariani, Z., Moeini, R.,
Shirafkan, H., & Amiri, M. (2020). Evaluation of the effect of *Silybum*
marianum extract on menopausal symptoms: A randomized, double-blind
placebo-controlled trial. *Phytotherapy Research, 34*(12), 3359–3366.
https://doi.org/10.1002/ptr.6789

65 A small trial: Ataei-Almanghadim, K., Farshbaf-Khalili, A., Ostadra-
himi, A. R., Shaseb, E., & Mirghafourvand, M. (2020). The effect of
oral capsule of curcumin and vitamin E on the hot flashes and anxiety
in postmenopausal women: A triple blind randomised controlled trial.
Complementary Therapies in Medicine, 48, Article 102267. https://doi.org
/10.1016/j.ctim.2019.102267

66 if CBD can keep you: Blessing, E. M., Steenkamp, M. M., Manzanares,
J., & Marmar, C. R. (2015). Cannabidiol as a potential treatment for
anxiety disorders. *Neurotherapeutics, 12*(4), 825–836. https://doi.org
/10.1007/s13311-015-0387-1

67 In a 2016 study: Bailey, T. G., Cable, N. T., Aziz, N., Dobson, R.,
Sprung, V. S., Low, D. A., & Jones, H. (2016). Exercise training reduces
the frequency of menopausal hot flushes by improving thermoregulatory
control. *Menopause, 23*(7), 708–718. https://doi.org/10.1097/gme
.0000000000000625

68 Research from the University of Maryland: Schilling, C., Gallicchio, L.,
Miller, S. R., Langenberg, P., Zacur, H., & Flaws, J. A. (2007). Current
alcohol use, hormone levels, and hot flashes in midlife women. *Fertility*
and Sterility, 87(6), 1483–1486. https://doi.org/10.1016/j.fertnstert
.2006.11.033

69 Research published in the journal: Avis, N. E., Coeytaux, R. R., Isom, S.,
Prevette, K., & Morgan, T. (2016). Acupuncture in Menopause (AIM)
study: A pragmatic, randomized controlled trial. *Menopause, 23*(6),
626–637. https://doi.org/10.1097/gme.0000000000000597

71 research suggests that: Price, M. (2011, March). *Placebos produce effect*

even when patients know it's just sugar. American Psychological Association. https://www.apa.org/monitor/2011/03/placebos

71 Dr. Wayne Jonas: Jonas, W. B. (2011). Reframing placebo in research and practice. *Philosophical Transactions of the Royal Society B: Biological Sciences, 366*(1572), 1896–1904. https://doi.org/10.1098/rstb.2010.0405

72 Robert Wood Johnson Medical School: Allen, L. A., Dobkin, R. D., Boohar, E. M., & Woolfolk, R. L. (2006). Cognitive behavior therapy for menopausal hot flashes: Two case reports. *Maturitas, 54*(1), 95–99. https://doi.org/10.1016/j.maturitas.2005.12.006

77 In one multicenter study: Moral, E., Delgado, J. L., Carmona, F., Caballero, B., Guillán, C., González, P. M., Suárez-Almarza, J., Velasco-Ortega, S., & Nieto, C. (2018). Genitourinary syndrome of menopause. Prevalence and quality of life in Spanish postmenopausal women. The GENISSE study. *Climacteric, 21*(2), 167–173. https://doi.org/10.1080/1 3697137.2017.1421921

78 Estrogen receptors . . . are present: Kim, H.-K., Kang, S.-Y., Chung, Y.-J., Kim, J.-H., & Kim, M.-R. (2015). The recent review of the genitourinary syndrome of menopause. *Journal of Menopausal Medicine, 21*(2), 65. https://doi.org/10.6118/jmm.2015.21.2.65

80 There are some interesting data: Amabebe, E., & Anumba, D. O. (2018). Psychosocial stress, cortisol levels, and maintenance of vaginal health. *Frontiers in Endocrinology, 9.* https://doi.org/10.3389/fendo.2018.00568

89 ACOG does recommend: American College of Obstetricians and Gynecologists. (n.d.). *The use of vaginal estrogen in women with a history of estrogen-dependent breast cancer.* https://www.acog.org/clinical/clinical -guidance/committee-opinion/articles/2016/03/the-use-of-vaginal -estrogen-in-women-with-a-history-of-estrogen-dependent-breast-cancer

91 Fat mass: Wu, B. N., & O'Sullivan, A. J. (2011). Sex differences in energy metabolism need to be considered with lifestyle modifications in humans. *Journal of Nutrition and Metabolism, 2011,* 1–6. https://doi.org /10.1155/2011/391809

92 our percentage of fat mass: Wu, B. N., & O'Sullivan, A. J. (2011). Sex differences in energy metabolism need to be considered with lifestyle modifications in humans. *Journal of Nutrition and Metabolism, 2011,* 1–6. https://doi.org/10.1155/2011/391809

92 In 2021, the journal *Science*: Pontzer, H., Yamada, Y., Sagayama, H., Ainslie, P. N., Andersen, L. F., Anderson, L. J., Arab, L., Baddou, I., Bedu-Addo, K., Blaak, E. E., Blanc, S., Bonomi, A. G., Bouten, C. V., Bovet, P., Buchowski, M. S., Butte, N. F., Camps, S. G., Close, G. L., Cooper, J. A., Speakman, J. R. (2021). Daily energy expenditure through the human life course. *Science, 373*(6556), 808–812. https://doi .org/10.1126/science.abe5017

93 the omentum: Meza-Perez, S., & Randall, T. D. (2017). Immunologi-

cal functions of the omentum. *Trends in Immunology*, *38*(7), 526–536. https://doi.org/10.1016/j.it.2017.03.002

96 "Embodiment theory": Frontiers. (n.d.). *Embodiment of emotion throughout the lifespan: The role of multi-modal processing in perception, cognition, action and social and emotional functioning.* https://www.frontiersin.org /research-topics/8911/embodiment-of-emotion-throughout-the-lifespan -the-role-of-multi-modal-processing-in-perception-cogni

98 "awkward, unattractive, ugly": Foster, G. D., Wadden, T. A., Makris, A. P., Davidson, D., Sanderson, R. S., Allison, D. B., & Kessler, A. (2003). Primary care physicians' attitudes about obesity and its treatment. *Obesity Research*, *11*(10), 1168–1177. https://doi.org/10.1038/oby.2003.161

102 you may start to notice: Thornton, J. (2007). Effect of estrogens on skin aging and the potential role of serums. *Clinical Interventions in Aging*, *2*(3): 283–297. https://doi.org/10.2147/cia.s798

107 up to two-thirds: Schwalfenberg, G. K., & Genuis, S. J. (2017). The importance of magnesium in clinical healthcare. *Scientifica*, *2017*, Article 4179326. https://doi.org/10.1155/2017/4179326

109 They come with: Johns Hopkins Lupus Center. (2019, March 27). *Osteoporosis medications (bisphosphonates).* https://www.hopkinslupus.org/lupus -treatment/common-medications-conditions/osteoporosis-medications -bisphosphonates/

110 impair the healthy functioning: Maltais, M. L., Desroches, J., & Dionne, I. J. (2009). Changes in muscle mass and strength after menopause. *Journal of Musculoskeletal and Neuronal Interactions*, *9*(4), 186–197. https:// pubmed.ncbi.nlm.nih.gov/19949277/

114 And in older people: Cannell, J. J., Hollis, B. W., Sorenson, M. B., Taft, T. N., & Anderson, J. J. B. (2009). Athletic performance and vitamin D. *Medicine & Science in Sports & Exercise*, *41*(5), 1102–1110. https://doi .org/10.1249/mss.0b013e3181930c2b

114 "indirectly exerts effects": Labrie, F., Luu-The, V., Bélanger, A., Lin, S.-X., Simard, J., Pelletier, G., & Labrie, C. (2005). Is dehydroepiandrosterone a hormone? *Journal of Endocrinology*, *187*(2), 169–196. https://doi.org /10.1677/joe.1.06264

115 However, the people: Bouchard, D. R., Soucy, L., Sénéchal, M., Dionne, I. J., & Brochu, M. (2009). Impact of resistance training with or without caloric restriction on physical capacity in obese older women. *Menopause*, *16*(1), 66–72. https://doi.org/10.1097/gme.0b013e31817dacf7

116 grams of protein: Gregorio, L., Brindisi, J., Kleppinger, A., Sullivan, R., Mangano, K. M., Bihuniak, J. D., Kenny, A. M., Kerstetter, J. E., & Insogn, K. L. (2013). Adequate dietary protein is associated with better physical performance among post-menopausal women 60–90 years. *The Journal of Nutrition, Health & Aging*, *18*(2), 155–160. https://doi.org/10 .1007/s12603-013-0391-2

118 In a study that included: Kwon, Y.-J., Lim, H.-J., Lee, Y.-J., Lee, H.-S., Linton, J. A., Lee, J. W., & Kang, H.-T. (2017). Associations between high-risk alcohol consumption and sarcopenia among postmenopausal women. *Menopause, 24*(9), 1022–1027. https://doi.org/10.1097/gme .0000000000000879

127 In fact, the organization: Baird, M. D., Zaber, M. A., Dick, A. W., Bird, C. E., Chen, A., Waymouth, M., Gahlon, G., Quigley, D. D., Al Ibrahim, H., & Frank, L. (2021, April). *The Wham Report: Societal impact of research funding for women's health in Alzheimer's disease and Alzheimer's disease–related dementias.* https://thewhamreport.org/wp-content/uploads /2021/04/TheWHAMReport_ADRD.pdf

127 "sex-specific cognitive reserve": Sundermann, E. E., Maki, P. M., Rubin, L. H., Lipton, R. B., Landau, S., & Biegon, A. (2016). Female advantage in verbal memory: Evidence of sex-specific cognitive reserve. *Neurology, 87*(18), 1916–1924. https://doi.org/10.1212/wnl.0000000000003288

128 glucose for energy: Chew, H., Solomon, V. A., & Fonteh, A. N. (2020). Involvement of lipids in Alzheimer's disease pathology and potential therapies. *Frontiers in Physiology, 11.* https://doi.org/10.3389/fphys.2020 .00598

Chapter 4: The Mind-Body Connection

147 ob-gyns can play: Bhat, A., Reed, S. D., & Unützer, J. (2017). The obstetrician-gynecologist's role in detecting, preventing, and treating depression. *Obstetrics & Gynecology, 129*(1), 157–163. https://doi.org /10.1097/aog.0000000000001809

Chapter 5: Physical Foundations of Mental Health

153 an unusually long-term: Freeman, E. W., & Sammel, M. D. (2016). Anxiety as a risk factor for menopausal hot flashes: Evidence from the Penn Ovarian Aging cohort. *Menopause, 23*(9), 942–949. https://doi.org /10.1097/gme.0000000000000662

154 For instance, a paper in *Menopause*: Elkins, G. R., Fisher, W. I., Johnson, A. K., Carpenter, J. S., & Keith, T. Z. (2013). Clinical hypnosis in the treatment of postmenopausal hot flashes. *Menopause, 20*(3), 291–298. https://doi.org/10.1097/gme.0b013e31826ce3ed

154 And a study from King's College London: Norton, S., Chilcot, J., & Hunter, M. S. (2014). Cognitive-behavior therapy for menopausal symptoms (hot flushes and night sweats). *Menopause, 21*(6), 574–578. https:// doi.org/10.1097/gme.0000000000000095

155 A landmark 2018 study: Koebele, S. V., Palmer, J. M., Hadder, B., Melikian, R., Fox, C., Strouse, I. M., DeNardo, D. F., George, C., Daunis, E., Nimer, A., Mayer, L. P., Dyer, C. A., & Bimonte-Nelson, H. A. (2018).

Hysterectomy uniquely impacts spatial memory in a rat model: A role for the nonpregnant uterus in cognitive processes. *Endocrinology, 160*(1), 1–19. https://doi.org/10.1210/en.2018-00709

158 Research from the Pennsylvania State University: Elavsky, S., & McAuley, E. (2007). Physical activity and mental health outcomes during menopause: A randomized controlled trial. *Annals of Behavioral Medicine, 33*(2), 132–142. https://doi.org/10.1007/bf02879894

158 A small study: Park, B. J., Tsunetsugu, Y., Kasetani, T., Kagawa, T., & Miyazaki, Y. (2009). The physiological effects of *Shinrin-yoku* (taking in the forest atmosphere or forest bathing): Evidence from field experiments in 24 forests across Japan. *Environmental Health and Preventive Medicine, 15*(1), 18–26. https://doi.org/10.1007/s12199-009-0086-9

159 A study done several years later: Song, C., Ikei, H., Park, B.-J., Lee, J., Kagawa, T., & Miyazaki, Y. (2018). Psychological benefits of walking through forest areas. *International Journal of Environmental Research and Public Health, 15*(12), 2804. https://doi.org/10.3390/ijerph15122804

159 boosts the immune system: Li, Q., Nakadai, A., Matsushima, H., Miyazaki, Y., Krensky, A. M., Kawada, T., & Morimoto, K. (2006). Phytoncides (wood essential oils) induce human natural killer cell activity. *Immunopharmacology and Immunotoxicology, 28*(2), 319–333. https://doi.org/10.1080/08923970600809439

159 improves blood glucose levels: Ohtsuka, Y., Yabunaka, N., & Takayama, S. (1998). Shinrin-yoku (forest-air bathing and walking) effectively decreases blood glucose levels in diabetic patients. *International Journal of Biometeorology, 41*(3), 125–127. https://doi.org/10.1007/s004840050064

159 may help fight cancer: Li, Q., Morimoto, K., Nakadai, A., Inagaki, H., Katsumata, M., Shimizu, T., Hirata, Y., Hirata, K., Suzuki, H., Miyazaki, Y., Kagawa, T., Koyama, Y., Ohira, T., Takayama, N., Krensky, A. M., & Kawada, T. (2007). Forest bathing enhances human natural killer activity and expression of anti-cancer proteins. *International Journal of Immunopathology and Pharmacology, 20*(2, Suppl.), S3–S8. https://doi.org/10.1177/03946320070200s202

159 can restore focus: Berman, M. G., Jonides, J., & Kaplan, S. (2008). The cognitive benefits of interacting with nature. *Psychological Science, 19*(12), 1207–1212. https://doi.org/10.1111/j.1467-9280.2008.02225.x

159 can help people with sleep problems: Morita, E., Imai, M., Okawa, M., Miyaura, T., & Miyazaki, S. (2011). A before and after comparison of the effects of forest walking on the sleep of a community-based sample of people with sleep complaints. *BioPsychoSocial Medicine, 5*(1), 13. https://doi.org/10.1186/1751-0759-5-13

160 the amount of greenness available: Casey, J., James, P., Cushing, L., Jesdale, B., & Morello-Frosch, R. (2017). Race, ethnicity, income concentration and 10-year change in urban greenness in the United States.

International Journal of Environmental Research and Public Health, *14*(12), 1546. https://doi.org/10.3390/ijerph14121546

161 Take exercise's effect on your brain: Barella, L. A., Etnier, J. L., & Chang, Y.-K. (2010). The immediate and delayed effects of an acute bout of exercise on cognitive performance of healthy older adults. *Journal of Aging and Physical Activity*, *18*(1), 87–98. https://doi.org/10.1123/japa.18.1.87

161 Even one session of weight training: Devereux, G. R., Wiles, J. D., & Howden, R. (2014). Immediate post-isometric exercise cardiovascular responses are associated with training-induced resting systolic blood pressure reductions. *European Journal of Applied Physiology*, *115*(2), 327–333. https://doi.org/10.1007/s00421-014-3021-8

161 a review of research: Friedenreich, C. M. (2004). Physical activity and breast cancer risk: The effect of menopausal status. *Exercise and Sport Sciences Reviews*, *32*(4), 180–184. https://doi.org/10.1097/00003677-200410000-00010

161 An interesting study: Schaafsma, M., Homewood, J., & Taylor, A. (2010). Subjective cognitive complaints at menopause associated with declines in performance of verbal memory and attentional processes. *Climacteric*, *13*(1), 84–98. https://doi.org/10.3109/13697130903009187

162 For instance, a study found: Maki, P. M., Springer, G., Anastos, K., Gustafson, D. R., Weber, K., Vance, D., Dykxhoorn, D., Milam, J., Adimora, A. A., Kassaye, S. G., Waldrop, D., & Rubin, L. H. (2021). Cognitive changes during the menopausal transition: A longitudinal study in women with and without HIV. *Menopause*, *28*(4), 360–368. https://doi.org/10.1097/gme.0000000000001725

162 A review of research: Sliwinski, J. R., Johnson, A. K., & Elkins, G. R. (2014). Memory decline in peri- and post-menopausal women: The potential of mind-body medicine to improve cognitive performance. *Integrative Medicine Insights*, *9*, 17–23. https://doi.org/10.4137/imi.s15682

163 Focus on berries: Spencer, J. P. (2009). Flavonoids and brain health: Multiple effects underpinned by common mechanisms. *Genes & Nutrition*, *4*(4), 243–250. https://doi.org/10.1007/s12263-009-0136-3

163 According to the National Institute on Aging: National Institute on Aging. (2019, April 23). *Social isolation, loneliness in older people pose health risks*. https://www.nia.nih.gov/news/social-isolation-loneliness-older-people-pose-health-risks

164 A paper written by: Carter, S., Jay, O., & Black, K. I. (2021). Talking about menopause in the workplace. *Case Reports in Women's Health*, *30*, Article e00306. https://doi.org/10.1016/j.crwh.2021.e00306

164 "menopausal status was not": Hardy, C., Thorne, E., Griffiths, A., &

Hunter, M. S. (2018, April 9). Work outcomes in midlife women: the impact of menopause, work stress and working environment. *Women's Midlife Health*, *4*, Article 3. https://doi.org/10.1186/s40695-018-00 36-z

165 In 2017, its Department for Education: Brewis, J., Beck, V., Davies, A., & Matheson, J. (1970, January 1). *The effects of menopause transition on women's economic participation in the UK*. Open Research Online. http://oro.open.ac.uk/59639/

168 A study by the RAND Corporation: Pollard, M. S., Tucker, J. S., & Green, H. D. (2020, September 29). Changes in adult alcohol use and consequences during the COVID-19 pandemic in the US. *JAMA Network Open*, *3*(9), Article e2022942. https://doi.org/10.1001/jamanet workopen.2020.22942

169 Research published in 2019: Sood, R., Kuhle, C. L., Kapoor, E., Thielen, J. M., Frohmader, K. S., Mara, K. C., & Faubion, S. S. (2019). Association of mindfulness and stress with menopausal symptoms in midlife women. *Climacteric*, *22*(4), 377–382. https://doi.org/10.1080/13697137 .2018.1551344

169 Plus, practicing mindfulness: Jacobs, T. L., Shaver, P. R., Epel, E. S., Zanesco, A. P., Aichele, S. R., Bridwell, D. A., Rosenberg, E. L., King, B. G., MacLean, K. A., Sahdra, B. K., Kemeny, M. E., Ferrer, E., Wallace, B. A., & Saron, C. D. (2013). Self-reported mindfulness and cortisol during a Shamatha meditation retreat. *Health Psychology*, *32*(10), 1104–1109. https://doi.org/10.1037/a0031362

172 More recent research indicates: Diego, M. A., & Field, T. (2009). Moderate pressure massage elicits a parasympathetic nervous system response. *International Journal of Neuroscience*, *119*(5), 630–638. https://doi.org/10 .1080/00207450802329605

172 Some studies have looked: Sankaran, R., Kamath, R., Nambiar, V., & Kumar, A. (2019). A prospective study on the effects of Ayurvedic massage in post-stroke patients. *Journal of Ayurveda and Integrative Medicine*, *10*(2), 126–130. https://doi.org/10.1016/j.jaim.2018.02.137

Chapter 6: Menopause and Mood Disorders

175 Nine women became depressed: Schmidt, P. J., Haq, N., & Rubinow, D. R. (2004). A longitudinal evaluation of the relationship between reproductive status and mood in perimenopausal women. *American Journal of Psychiatry*, *161*(12), 2238–2244. https://doi.org/10.1176/appi.ajp.161.12 .2238

176 Amina Sboui: Jonathan Jones. (2013, April 5). A gloriously crude topless "jihad" from a Femen activist. *The Guardian*. https://www.theguardian .com/commentisfree/2013/apr/05/femen-topless-protest-gloriously-crude

Chapter 7: Prejudice in Medicine

183 "I was like, a Doppler?": Haskell, R. (2018, January 10). Serena Williams on motherhood, marriage, and making her comeback. *Vogue*. https:// www.vogue.com/article/serena-williams-vogue-cover-interview-february -2018

184 The quality of cardiac: Bridges, K. M. (n.d.). *Implicit bias and racial disparities in health care*. American Bar Association. https://www.american bar.org/groups/crsj/publications/human_rights_magazine_home/the -state-of-healthcare-in-the-united-states/racial-disparities-in-health-care/

184 "Black patients with heart disease": Bridges, K. M. (n.d.). *Implicit bias and racial disparities in health care*. American Bar Association. https:// www.americanbar.org/groups/crsj/publications/human_rights_magazine _home/the-state-of-healthcare-in-the-united-states/racial-disparities-in -health-care/

185 Socioeconomic realities and stress: Velez, A. (2021, March 10). *Menopause is different for women of color*. EndocrineWeb. https://www.endocrineweb .com/menopause-different-women-color

Chapter 8: Breaking Free from the Societal Bullshit

195 A study published in *Proceedings*: Nattrass, S., Croft, D. P., Ellis, S., Cant, M. A., Weiss, M. N., Wright, B. M., Stredulinsky, E., Doniol-Valcroze, T., Ford, J. K., Balcomb, K. C., & Franks, D. W. (2019). Postreproductive killer whale grandmothers improve the survival of their grandoffspring. *Proceedings of the National Academy of Sciences of the United States of America, 116*(52), 26669–26673. https://doi.org/10.1073/pnas.19038 44116

195 can increase cognitive development in children: Lee, H., Ryan, L. H., Ofstedal, M. B., & Smith, J. (2020). Multigenerational households during childhood and trajectories of cognitive functioning among U.S. older adults. *The Journals of Gerontology: Series B, 76*(6), 1161–1172. https://doi .org/10.1093/geronb/gbaa165

195 can reduce stress: Muennig, P., Jiao, B., & Singer, E. (2018). Living with parents or grandparents increases social capital and survival: 2014 General Social Survey—National Death Index. *SSM—Population Health, 4*, 71–75. https://doi.org/10.1016/j.ssmph.2017.11.001

195 Here are some: Seppala, E. (2017, June 28). *Connectedness & health: The science of social connection*. The Center for Compassion and Altruism Research and Education. http://ccare.stanford.edu/uncategorized /connectedness-health-the-science-of-social-connection-infographic/

197 Here's a fun little study: Cohen, S., Janicki-Deverts, D., Turner, R. B., & Doyle, W. J. (2014). Does hugging provide stress-buffering social support? A study of susceptibility to upper respiratory infection and illness.

Psychological Science, 26(2), 135–147. https://doi.org/10.1177/09567
97614559284
198 "Gratitude is a positive": Bartlett, M. Y., & Arpin, S. N. (2019). Gratitude and loneliness: Enhancing health and well-being in older adults. *Research on Aging, 41*(8), 772–793. https://doi.org/10.1177/0164
027519845354

Chapter 9: Eat for Health and Joy

217 Studies have shown: Stunkard, A. J., Harris, J. R., Pedersen, N. L., & McClearn, G. E. (1990). The body-mass index of twins who have been reared apart. *The New England Journal of Medicine, 322*(21), 1483–1487. https://doi.org/10.1056/nejm199005243222102
223 Strings told NPR: NPR. (2020, July 21). *Fat phobia and its racist past and present.* NPR. https://www.npr.org/transcripts/893006538
224 In fact, the human: Turnbaugh, P. J., Ley, R. E., Hamady, M., Fraser-Liggett, C. M., Knight, R., & Gordon, J. I. (2007). The Human Microbiome Project. *Nature, 449*(7164), 804–810. https://doi.org/10.1038
/nature06244
225 There's even something: Bodai, B. I., & Nakata, T. E. (2020). Breast cancer: Lifestyle, the human gut microbiota/microbiome, and survivorship. *The Permanente Journal, 24*(19), Article 129. https://doi.org/10.7812/tpp
/19.129
225 "Inside our bellies": Campos, M. (2021, November 16). *Leaky gut: What is it, and what does it mean for you?* Harvard Health. https://www.health
.harvard.edu/blog/leaky-gut-what-is-it-and-what-does-it-mean-for-you
-2017092212451
226 "When a high-fiber diet": Bodai, B. I., & Nakata, T. E. (2020). Breast cancer: Lifestyle, the human gut microbiota/microbiome, and survivorship. *The Permanente Journal, 24*(19), Article 129. https://doi.org/10
.7812/tpp/19.129

INDEX

Page numbers of illustrations appear in italics.

ABOUT THE AUTHOR

A Diplomat of the American College of Obstetrics and Gynecology, **Dr. Suzanne Gilberg-Lenz** received her medical degree in 1996 from the USC School of Medicine and completed her residency in obstetrics and gynecology at Cedars-Sinai Medical Center. Dr. Gilberg-Lenz is involved in women's empowerment and public education and appears frequently as an expert in women's health and integrative medicine on TV, in print, and online. She completed her clinical Ayurvedic Specialist degree at California College of Ayurveda in 2010 and was board-certified in integrative and holistic medicine in 2008. Dr. Gilberg-Lenz has appeared on *Today*; *CNN Headline News*; the *Steve Harvey Morning Show*; and the *Dr. Oz Show*. Dr. Gilberg-Lenz is cofounder of Cedars-Sinai Medical Center's Green Committee and is deeply committed to the promotion of healing that involves individuals, families, communities, and the planet.